the healthy
back

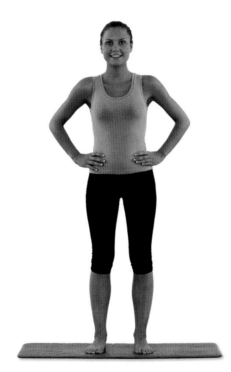

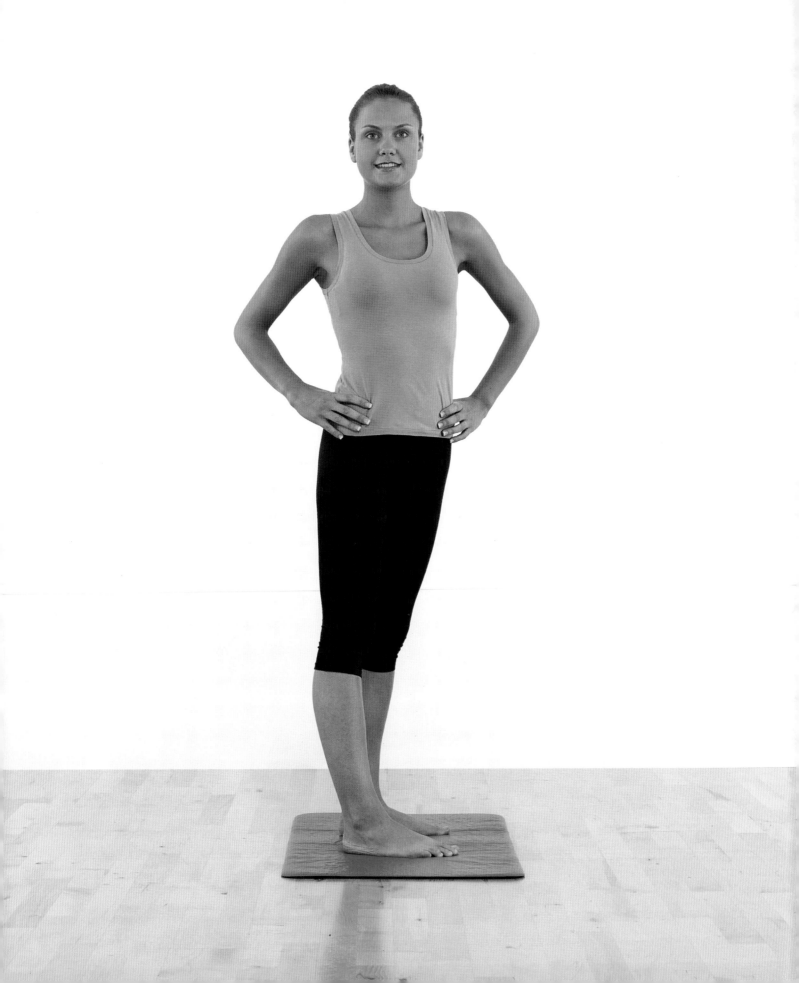

the healthy
back

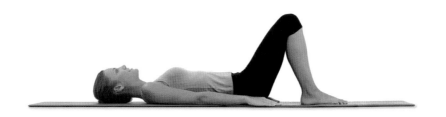

kim davies

p

This is a Parragon Publishing Book
First published in 2006

Parragon Publishing
Queen Street House
4 Queen Street
Bath BA1 1HE, UK

ISBN: 978-1-4054-8647-7
Printed in China

Created and produced by the Bridgewater Book Company Ltd
Photography: Ian Parsons
Hair and make-up stylist: Johan van der Merwe
Models: Sky Bliss and Emily Nelson

The publisher would like to thank the following for permission
to reproduce copyright material: **Corbis**/Artiga Photo: 40;
Emma Rian/zefa: 42; Jana Renee Cruder: 16 left; Jon Feingersh: 95;
Michael Keller: 25; Rob Lewine: 62; **Getty Images**/Anthony Nagelmenn/
Taxi: 25; Arthur Tilley/Stone: 23; Arthur Tilley/Taxi: 22; Barry Yee/
Photographer's Choice: 43; Brooke Fasani/Iconica: 78; David Joel/
Photographer's Choice: 93; Longview/The Image Bank: 26; Louis Fox/
Taxi: 16 right; Pierre Bourrier/Photonica: 80; Ryan McVay/The Image
Bank: 17; White Cross Productions/The Image Bank: 89; **iStockphoto**: 6,
12, 14, 21, 30, 76, 79 bottom, 81, 86; **Jupiter Images**: 24, 27.

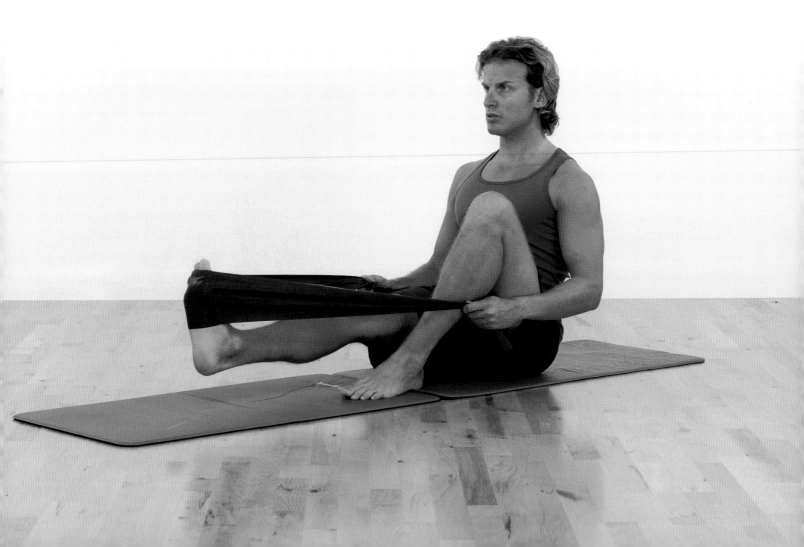

contents

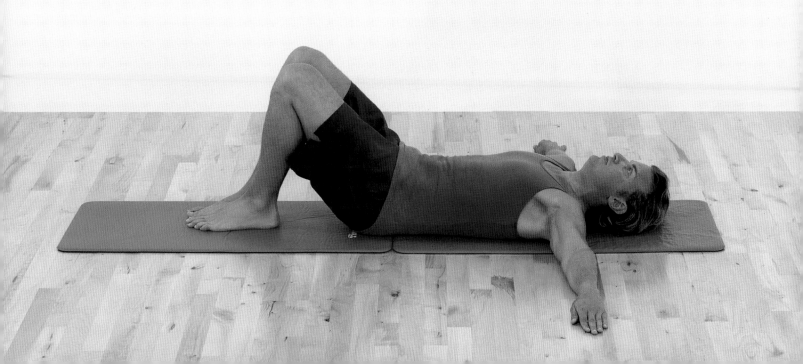

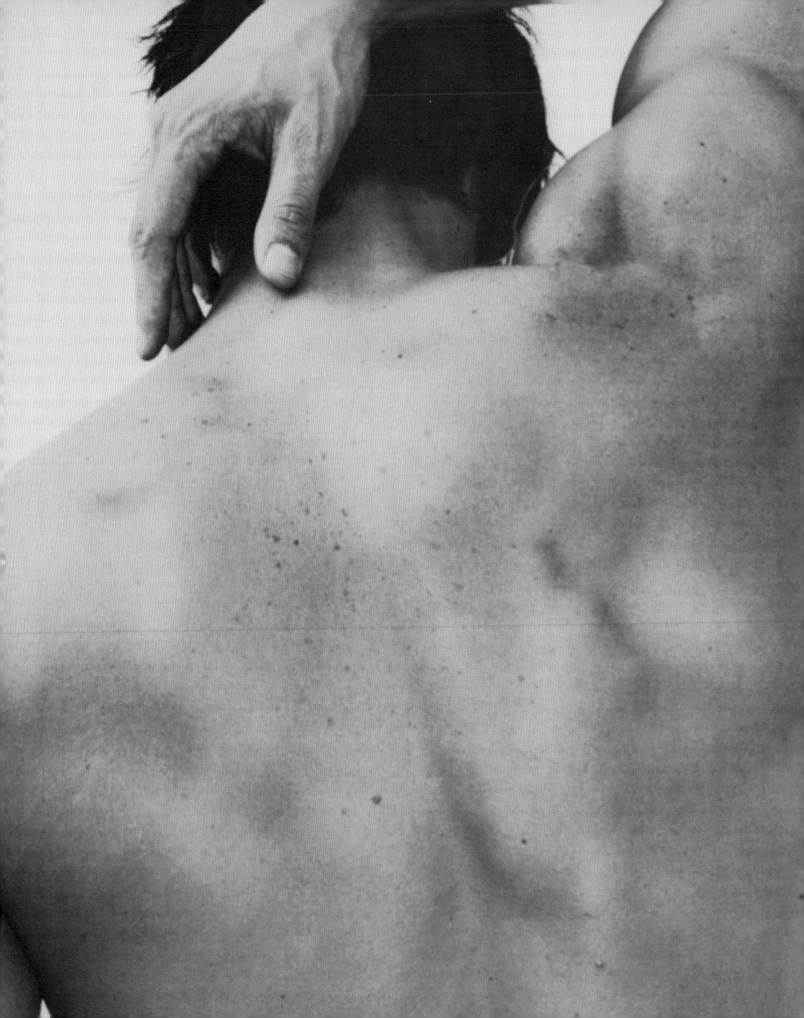

1. a healthy back

The spine is a real feat of mechanical engineering.
It enables us to walk upright, to bend over, to turn,
and to stretch. It supports the head and trunk, and is
involved in almost every movement that we make.
It also has a protective function, because it encases
the vulnerable central nervous system. But to do its
job properly, the spine needs support from the
muscles and ligaments of the back.

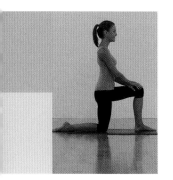

how the back works

The back is a complex structure of sturdy bones, strong muscles, and flexible ligaments and tendons overlaid with a dense network of nerves. All these need to be working in harmony in order to keep the back healthy.

the spine

The spine is made up of 33 irregularly shaped bones—the vertebrae. These bones are stacked on top of each other like a tower, and they are linked by small joints (facet joints) and strong ligaments. Thin rubbery disks act as shock absorbers between the main vertebrae.

A healthy adult spine is not ramrod-straight: it curves gently in, out, and in again, forming a shallow S-shape. This neutral alignment protects the spine from stress by helping to absorb reverberations through our bodies as we walk, run, and jump. There are five distinct regions of the spine. These are, from the top downward:

Cervical spine (neck) Seven vertebrae make up the cervical spine, which supports the head. They include the atlas and axis at the base of the head, which act like pivots, enabling the head to move freely up and down and from side to side.

Thoracic spine (upper back) There are 12 vertebrae in the upper back. They are anchored to the ribs, and so help to protect the heart and lungs. This extra attachment means that the upper back necessarily has less mobility than the neck and the lower back.

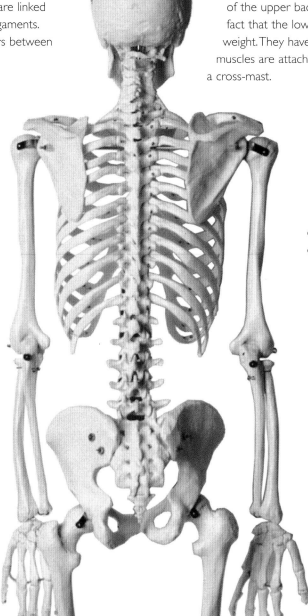

Lumbar spine (lower back) The five lumbar vertebrae are much larger and sturdier than those of the upper back and neck, to compensate for the fact that the lower back takes most of the body's weight. They have bony protrusions to which strong muscles are attached for extra support, like rigging on a cross-mast.

Sacrum and coccyx The sacrum consists of five vertebrae that are fused together. Four more tiny fused vertebrae make up the coccyx (tailbone). The sacrum helps to protect the reproductive organs and the bladder, while the coccyx is a vestige of the tail that our distant lemur-like ancestors used to help them swing through the trees. It has no function in modern humans.

a protective shell

The bones of the spine provide a protective casing for the spinal cord. This cord is essentially a biological cable of nerves, which acts as a kind of information highway. It runs from the base of the brain to the lumbar vertebrae. Nerves pass from the spinal cord through gaps in each vertebra to carry messages to all parts of the body. The spinal cord is bathed in cerebrospinal fluid and encased in three layers of membrane. The casing is highly elastic, so that the spinal cord can bend with the spine.

intervertebral disks

The oval-shaped disks that separate the main vertebrae are shock absorbers, which protect the bones of the spine from sudden impact, weight, and pressure. They have a tough outer skin (annular), which contains a jelly-like substance (the nucleus). This means that they change shape when placed under pressure—if you bend forward, for example, the front of the intervertebral disks will flatten and the back will expand. This pliability is what allows the spine most of its movement.

During the course of a day, pressure on the intervertebral disks means that some of the water content in the nucleus leaches out into the surrounding soft tissues, and so the disks become slightly thinner. At night, when you are lying down, the pressure is taken off and the water content is replenished. As a result, the average person is about ½ in (1 cm) taller in the morning than in the evening. Over a lifetime, some of the water content is lost from the disk for good—which is why you can be ½–2 in (1–5 cm) shorter in old age.

inside a vertebra...

The small facet joints and the intervertebral disks between each vertebra work together to enable the spine to twist and bend. The ligaments and muscles—attached to bony protrusions called vertebral processes—serve to support and stabilize the spine. The muscles also constitute an ingenious pulley system, which enables the back to move in a controlled way.

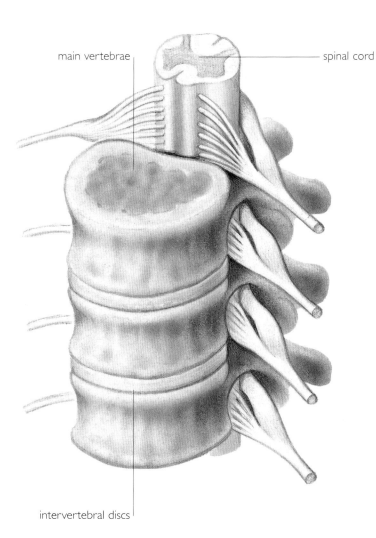

main vertebrae

spinal cord

intervertebral discs

facet joints

Each vertebra has two pairs of bony extensions, called facet joints, which link it with its neighbors. Each joint is covered with cartilage, which gives a smooth surface and so enables the protrusions to glide easily over each other. This helps to facilitate the forward and backward movements of the spine.

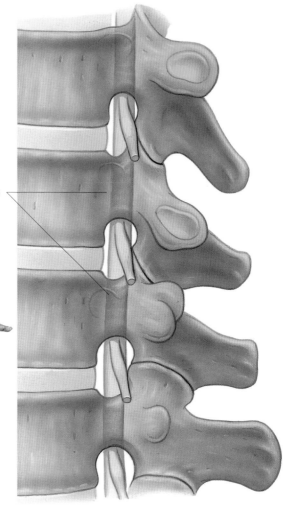

facet joints

ligaments

Ligaments are tough bands of fibrous tissue that connect two bones and help to stabilize a joint. In the back, small ligaments connect the vertebrae and larger ligaments run between groups of vertebrae.

Ligaments limit movement, which helps to protect the joints from injury. A ligament that is underused becomes stiff and makes movement more difficult, while a ligament that is frequently overstretched will become slack and lose its ability to limit excessive movement.

muscles

Muscles power movement and help to maintain posture. They are connected to bones either directly or by bands of strong tissue (tendons) and are usually arranged in pairs, one on either side of a joint. As the muscle on one side contracts, the corresponding muscle on the other side lengthens, enabling the bone or joint to move. It is exactly the same principle as is used in a mechanical winch or crane.

The muscles of the back are arranged in several layers. The superficial muscles, which are closest to the skin's surface, are mainly broad sheets of muscles that connect the vertebrae to the shoulder blades and joints. The middle layer consists of strap-shaped muscles that run over the lower ribs, chest, and lower back. The deepest muscles run from one vertebra to another, helping to keep them in position.

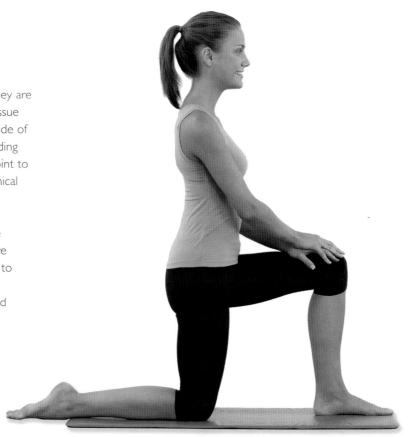

The abdominal muscles work in tandem with the muscles of the back to support and stabilize the spine. When contracted, they increase the pressure in the abdominal cavity, which reduces stress on the spine. Also important are the hip flexors (psoas), which run from the upper part of the thigh bone to the lumbar vertebrae, and the hamstrings. Inflexible hip flexors and leg muscles increase the pressure on the back muscles, making back pain or stiffness more likely.

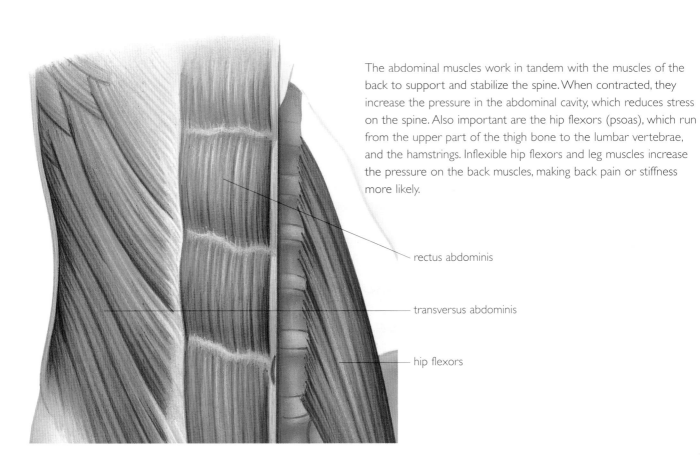

rectus abdominis

transversus abdominis

hip flexors

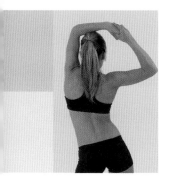

how the back moves

To keep the back healthy and enable it to perform a full range of movements, three things are necessary: mobility of the spine, supple muscles, and strength. All these can be achieved by doing moderate exercise regularly and correctly.

Doing specific back exercises in addition to exercise such as swimming or brisk walking will help to ensure that you are working all the important muscle groups. Regular movement helps to maintain the elasticity of the muscles and it builds their power. It also serves to keep the joints mobile. Movement encourages good circulation of blood and other fluids around the body. This helps to keep the joints lubricated and enables muscles and joints to take in nutrients and to expel waste products.

It's important to hold the body correctly when you are exercising and when you are going about your normal day's activities. If the body is held in an abnormal way or you perform an awkward movement, then excessive strain is placed on the joints. This is as true for people who are superfit as it is for those who don't exercise enough. Dancers and yoga practitioners can develop excessive mobility in their joints as a result of performing an outlandish range of movements. This is like driving without brakes—the muscles' inbuilt safety mechanisms are not functioning. Mobility needs to be complemented with stability in order to protect the back.

A key to maintaining stability in the back is the correct use of the deepest abdominal muscle—the transversus abdominis. This muscle is just below your navel and runs in a band from one side of the abdomen to the other. When you contract this muscle, it takes the pressure off the spine. A body builder will instinctively pull in this muscle before lifting a heavy weight. Learning how to use this muscle properly is an important element of back care.

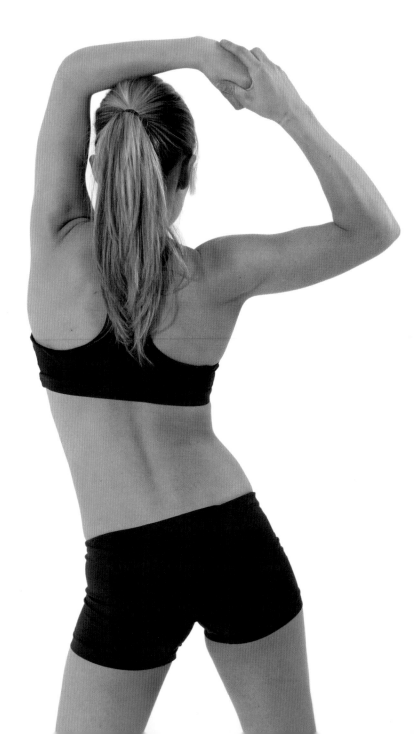

movements of the back

All back movements involve one or more of four basic movements: rotation, flexion, side flexion, or extension. The muscles of the back, legs, hips, and abdomen are all involved in these everyday movements.

rotation

BELOW Muscles at the side of the spine are used to twist the trunk to the side. This movement enables you to turn around while sitting or standing.

extension

BELOW Extension is bending backward. It involves the long muscles that go down the spine (erector spinae) and also the muscles of the buttocks and abdomen.

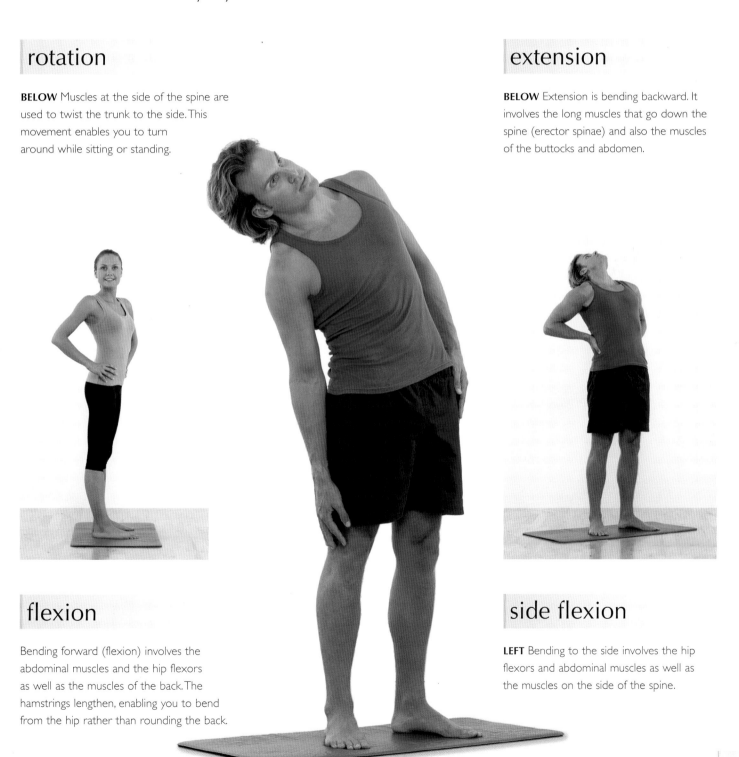

flexion

Bending forward (flexion) involves the abdominal muscles and the hip flexors as well as the muscles of the back. The hamstrings lengthen, enabling you to bend from the hip rather than rounding the back.

side flexion

LEFT Bending to the side involves the hip flexors and abdominal muscles as well as the muscles on the side of the spine.

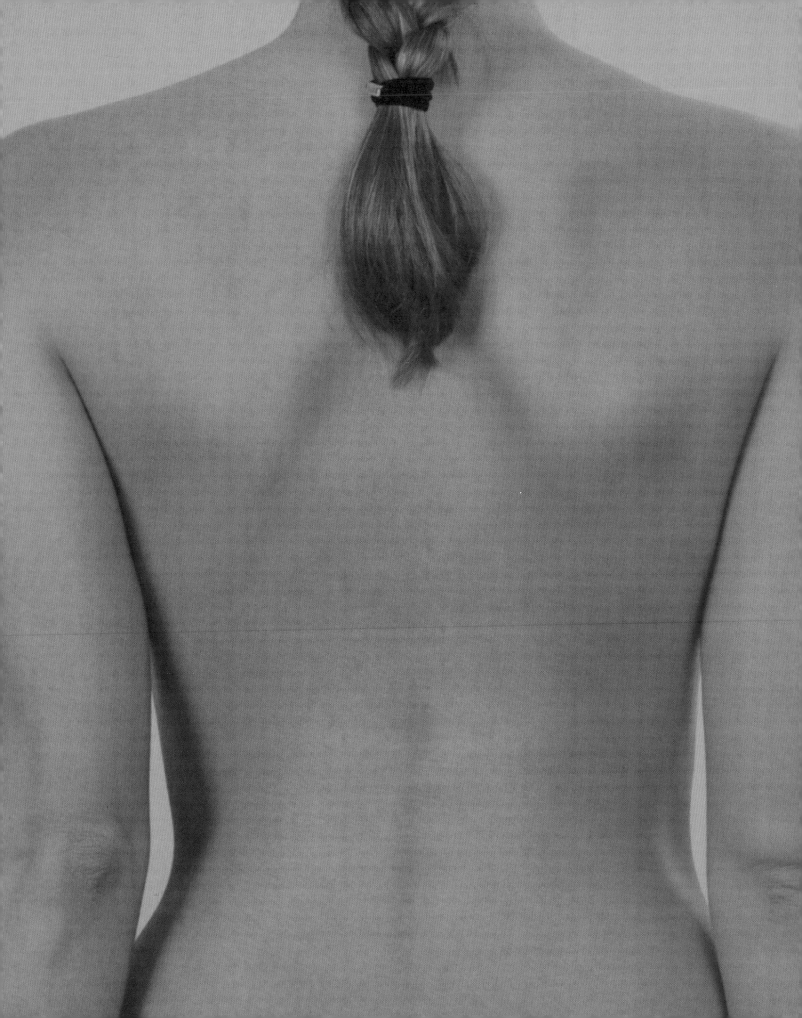

2. keeping your back in good working order

Maintaining good posture is the single best thing you can do to help keep your back healthy. Keeping generally fit and active and doing regular back exercises will go a long way toward achieving good posture. But it is also important to build awareness of the way you hold yourself during your everyday activities. Get into the habit of stopping what you are doing at regular intervals and think about how you are standing or sitting. Move to relieve any discomfort and take a few deep breaths to relax.

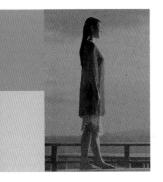

posture

The best way to keep your back healthy is to maintain an erect but natural posture at all times.

recognizing poor posture

At first, maintaining an erect, natural posture requires constant attention. When you stand or sit well, your muscles are balanced and relaxed and minimal strain is placed on the joints and ligaments. When you sit or stand awkwardly, the muscles, joints, and ligaments are put under pressure. Over time, this can lead to back problems.

Poor posture develops over a long period. It can also become such a habit that standing or sitting badly starts to feel normal. As a result, it may feel odd or uncomfortable when you do stand properly. Recognizing poor posture is the first step to improving it.

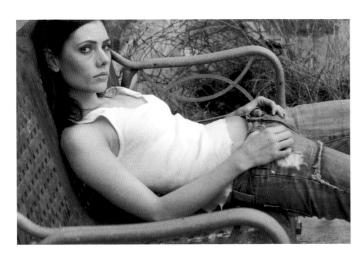

swayback

ABOVE The most common form of poor posture is slouching, which is known as swayback. The muscles become loose, they stop holding the back so tightly, and the curves of the spine are exaggerated. People who are overweight are prone to slouching.

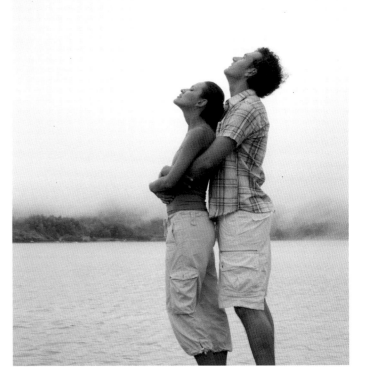

flat back

ABOVE Standing too straight can be just as damaging to the back as slouching, since it constricts the muscles and makes deep breathing difficult. Over time, the back becomes straighter, which increases pressure on the spine.

good posture

BELOW When you hold yourself well, your body weight is distributed evenly and all your joints are held in a neutral position that places minimum strain on them. The muscles are well balanced and relaxed, and the stomach, lungs, and other organs are free of any constriction.

tips for posture...

- Avoid standing or sitting for long periods—take a break at least once an hour.
- When standing, always spread your weight between both feet.
- Do not wear high heels, which throw the pelvis and spine out of line.

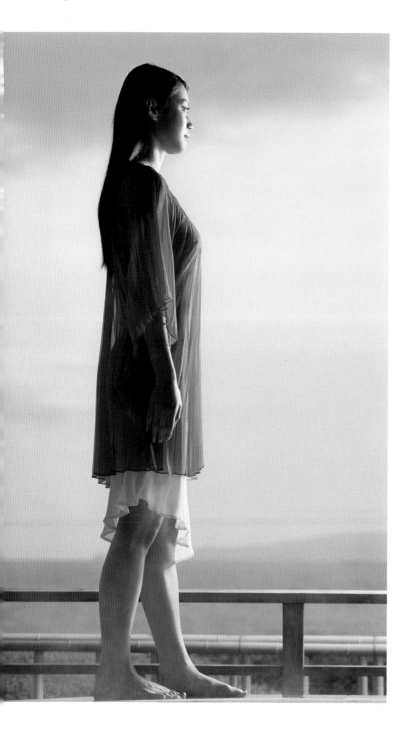
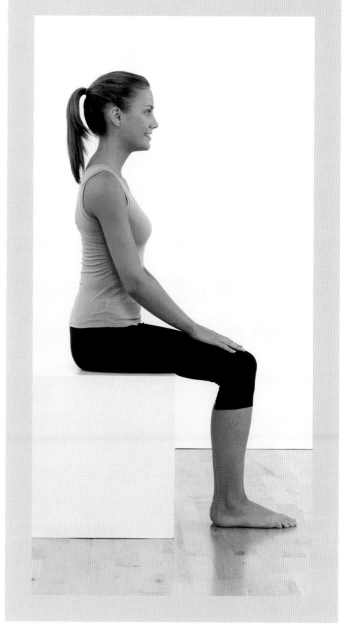

improving your posture

This is a quick exercise that you can do at any time of day to pull yourself up straight. It can help to do it in front of a mirror from time to time.

step 1

BELOW Stand tall with your feet pointing forward, about hip-width apart. Place your hands on your hips. Slowly bring your weight onto your heels, but leave the balls of your feet on the floor. Then bring your weight onto the balls of your feet, leaving your heels on the floor. Now raise your toes from the floor: this should distribute your weight evenly between balls and heels. Bring the toes back to the floor.

step 3

BELOW Then push your hips forward, so that your bottom comes in and your pelvis tips backward.

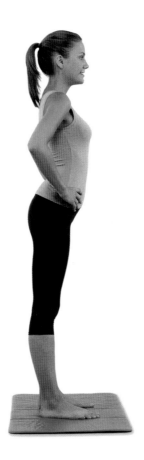

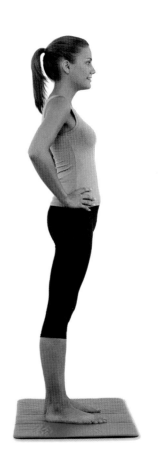

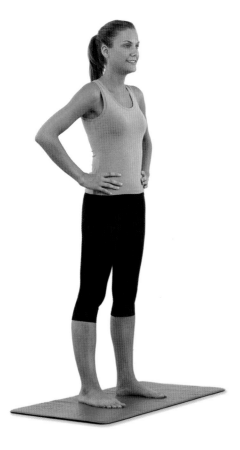

step 2

ABOVE Place your hands on your hips. Stick your bottom out so that your pelvis tips forward.

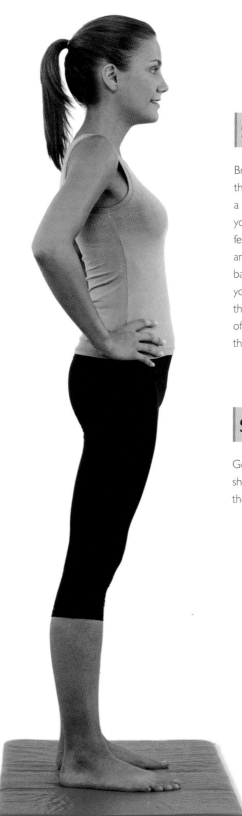

step 4

Find the midway point between these two positions: this is the neutral position for the pelvis. Pull up on your pelvic floor muscles and draw in the abdomen: this helps you to maintain the pelvis in neutral.

step 5

Bring your shoulders up toward your ears and hold for a moment, then let them drop. Bring them forward, rounding the upper back and compressing the chest. Hold for a moment and then pull them backward, drawing the shoulder blades toward each other and down your back. Relax: your shoulders should stay back and down.

tip...

Keep your knees "soft" rather than locked. To stand up straight, pull up on the thigh muscles rather than pushing the knees back.

step 6

Bring your head up, so that it is in line with the spine. It helps to imagine that there is a piece of string attached to the crown of your head; you can pull on a few hairs to feel the effect of this. Raise your chin upward and notice how the crown of your head tilts backward. Then drop the chin; the crown of your head drops forward. Bring the head into the midway, neutral position so that the top of the head and the chin are parallel with the floor.

step 7

Go through the main points again: feet, pelvis, shoulders, and head, checking that each is in the right position.

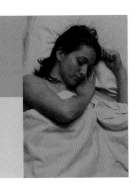

sleeping

A good night's sleep is an essential part of back care. Not only does deep rest let your muscles relax, but lying down relieves pressure on the intervertebral disks, enabling them to spring back into shape.

the perfect bed

Lots of people wake up feeling stiff and aching because they are sleeping on the wrong mattress, such as one that sags or is overly hard. When buying a bed, consider the following points:

- Choose a bed with a finely sprung mattress. If you sleep on your side, make sure that there is enough "give" to enable the hips and shoulders to sink into the mattress slightly so that the spine stays in alignment.

- Make sure that the bed feels comfortable for you: lie on it in your usual sleeping position for as long as possible to get an idea.

- Choose a base that is firm or slatted. A bed base that sags or is springy can be harmful to your back and reduce the lifespan of your mattress.

- Check that the bed is long enough for you: a good bed should be at least 6 in (15 cm) longer than your height to enable you to move around comfortably.

- Choose a bed that you can get in and out of easily, so not too high or low.

- If you are sharing the bed, make sure that it is wide enough to suit you both. You should both lie on it at the same time to check, and to ensure that it is equally wide for both of you. If not, consider pushing twin beds together.

what pillow?

When you rest at night, you want to be in a position that keeps your spine as straight as possible. Using lots of pillows will push your neck out of alignment with the rest of the spine. If you lie on your back, you may not need a pillow. One pillow is usually sufficient to keep the spine in line if you are sleeping on your side, but some people need two. A special neck-support pillow is higher at the front to keep the neck in a good position; if you are using an ordinary pillow, push it well into the shoulder for a similar effect.

- Most people find lying on their side most comfortable. Placing a pillow between the knees helps to prevent the spine from twisting.

- If you lie on your back, try placing a pillow under your knees to reduce any strain on the lower back.

- Lying on your stomach means twisting your neck to one side or the other, so it is not a good position to sleep in. Placing pillows under one hip and leg can improve the alignment of the spine.

tip...

If you have a springy bed base, try putting a board under the mattress. It should be cut to the same size as the base and be thick enough not to bend under your weight—a board ¾ in (2 cm) thick is sufficient for most people.

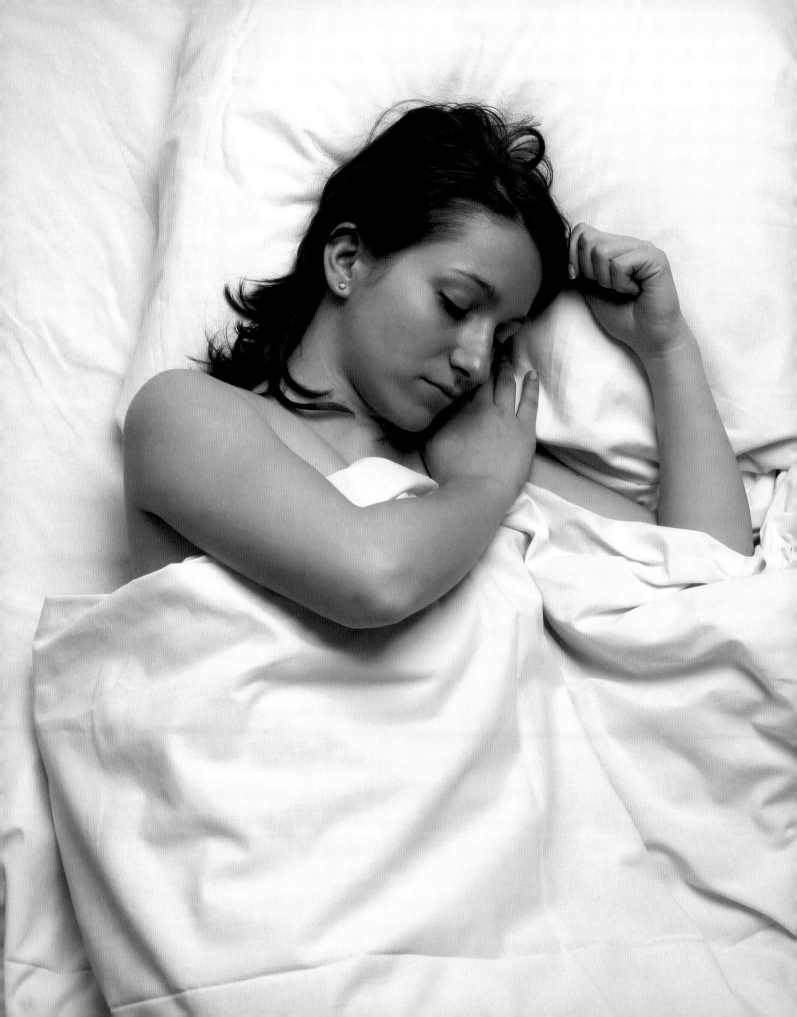

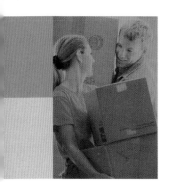

lifting

Not knowing the correct way to lift heavy objects is one of the most common causes of strained backs. All of us lift up objects throughout our daily routines, so learning good lifting techniques is a simple way of helping you keep a healthy back.

lifting a heavy item

If you need to lift a heavy object, you must do it in a way that minimizes the strain on the back by using your leg muscles to take the weight, rather than stooping over.

step 1

Stand directly in front of the object. Bend your knees in order to reach it, keeping your back straight (do not bend from the waist). You want to get as close as you can, with your knees on either side of the object. Your feet should be parallel to each other (both pointing outward). If possible, face the direction that you are going to move in.

step 2

Put one hand underneath the object and use the other to steady it. Lean forward so that your back is inclined toward the object but remains straight.

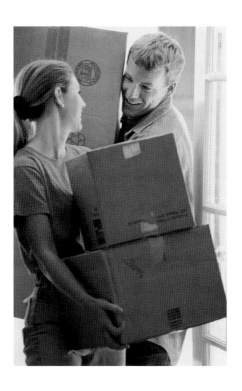

step 3

Stand up in one smooth, slow movement, keeping the object close to your body and taking your weight on your legs. Do not round your back as you come up.

step 4

Wait until you are standing completely upright before turning the whole body in the direction you wish to move in. Put the object down in the same way as you lifted it.

tips for lifting...

- Keep the burden balanced. If you are carrying heavy shopping, for example, divide it between two bags of equal weight, and carry one in each hand. Use a backpack rather than a heavy shoulder bag.
- Never try to lift something that is too heavy for you. Get someone else to help.
- Always position yourself so that the thing you are lifting is in front of you, not at your side. Do not twist around and then pick something up—even something as light as a book.
- Keep the object close to you as you move.
- Don't lift a heavy object above your head.

lifting children

If you have young children, you will be doing a lot of lifting and carrying. Use the basic principles for lifting any heavy weight in order to protect your back as much as possible.

step 1

Always stand in front of a toddler and squat before picking him or her up.

step 2

Put both hands under the child's arms in order to lift him or her up.

tips for lifting...

- Buy a crib with a drop-down side to reduce the amount you have to bend over to pick up your child.
- Once a child is old enough to stand, get him or her to do so before lifting.
- Take special care to avoid making twisting movements as, say, you lift your toddler out of his or her car seat.
- Don't change your baby on the floor. Invest in a changing table for diaper-changing, or use a chest of drawers at the right height.
- Remember that the ligaments stretch during pregnancy and take several months to return to normal. Take extra care to avoid straining your back at this time.
- If you are breastfeeding, use cushions to raise the baby up to the level of your breast.

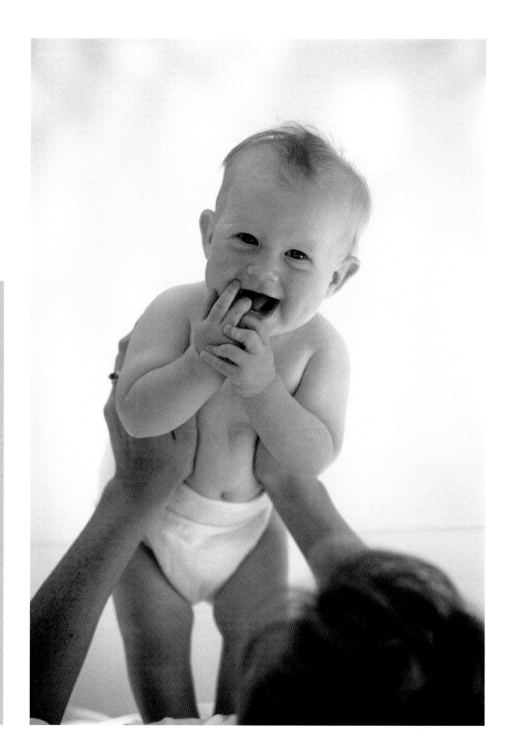

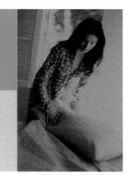

gardening and housework

Many everyday tasks in the garden and home involve repetitive bending and lifting movements. Taking a few precautionary measures will help reduce any strain on your back.

safe digging

Rest the spade on the ground and then use your body weight to push the blade into the earth. Keep your feet at a comfortable distance apart, and hold the spade firmly but not tightly, to avoid tensing the arm and shoulder muscles.

Press the blade into each side of the spadeful, so that the earth has been loosened on three sides. Then bend your knees and grasp the base of the handle to lever out the earth. Lift the blade and turn it over to drop the soil. Don't try to lift a large amount of soil in one go.

tips for gardeners...

- Always warm up before gardening by doing some brisk walking on the spot and a few simple stretches.
- Vary your activities so that you don't spend a whole day digging or bending over to weed. Take lots of breaks.
- Avoid kneeling as much as possible. To weed, try squatting with one knee on the ground, and then change legs every couple of minutes. Use a kneeling mat or knee pads.
- Use long-handled tools wherever you can.
- When mowing, be sure to keep your back straight rather than leaning forward.
- Fill a wheelbarrow with a small load only. Where possible, bag trash up rather than filling a wheelbarrow.
- Work in the afternoons rather than mornings because you are less stiff at this time of day.
- Don't try to dig ground that is very wet.

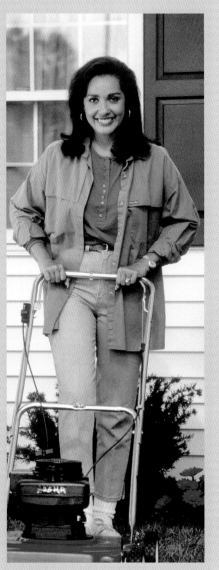

ironing

Set the ironing board at a height so that you do not have to stoop, but make sure that your arm is comfortable—your elbow should be at an angle of about 90°. Placing one foot on a low step or a block will help to relieve the strain on your back if you have to iron a lot of items in one go—but ideally iron little and often.

washing clothes

Squat or kneel to get washing in or out of a machine rather than bending over. Remember that wet washing is heavy—put a few clothes in a laundry basket at a time rather than trying to lift a whole load in one go. Keep the washing line at a reasonable height so that you don't have to strain to hang washing out.

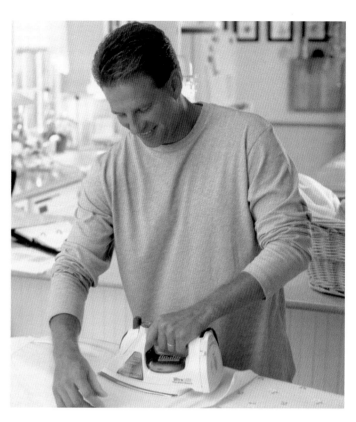

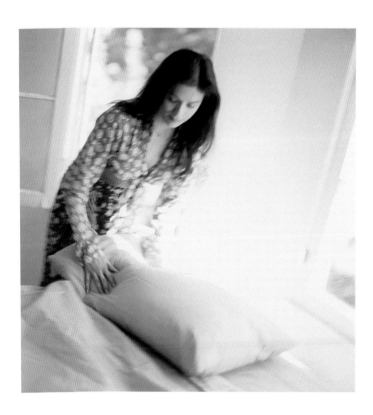

cleaning

Use an upright vacuum cleaner and keep it close to your body to reduce any strain on your back. Kneel or squat to clean the bath or baseboards so that you can keep your back straight. Make sure you kneel on a mat rather than a hard floor.

bedmaking

Use fitted sheets and a duvet, which are less effort to make up than flat sheets and blankets. Squat or kneel down to tuck sheets in rather than stooping over.

tips for doing housework...

Do some simple stretches before starting housework. Vary your activities as much as possible so that you don't spend long periods in one position: for example, vacuum and then dust a room rather than vacuuming your whole home in one go.

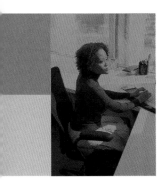

how to sit

Many back problems have their roots in the sedentary lifestyles most of us lead. Sitting is much harder on the spine than lying down or standing, especially if you also slouch or lean forward.

Everyone relaxes their posture when they sit down. But many chairs seem almost designed to force your spine into the slouchiest position possible. To protect your spine, it is a good idea to avoid sitting on a very soft armchair or on a very low chair that pushes the thighs higher than the hips. Try not to sit in the same position for long periods—a rocking chair is good because it naturally encourages you to keep changing position.

working at a desk

If you work sitting down, then it is essential to have a good chair that you can adjust to suit your individual needs. This is what you need from an office chair.

- Computer set level with the eyes so that head can be held erect.

- Back support to help maintain the natural curves of the spine.

- Deep seat that supports the legs as far as the knee joints.

- Seat at a height that enables your thighs to be level with the floor and your lower legs to be at right angles to your feet. The feet should be firmly on the floor or on a low block.

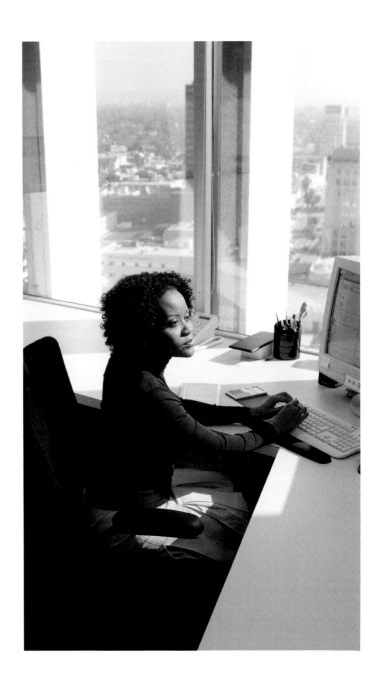

comfortable driving

Driving for long periods increases the risk of back pain: people who drive for more than four hours a day are six times more likely to take time off work for back pain than those who drive for two hours or less.

When you are driving, the body is confined in a fixed position, and it is subject to vibration and movement. The feet are manipulating the pedals, so they cannot help to stabilize the lower back as they do when you are sitting on a chair. The following may help you:

● Adjust the height of the seat so that you can comfortably reach the pedals and your thighs are parallel with the floor.

● Check that you can reach the steering wheel easily. Your arms should remain slightly bent.

● Make sure that you can rest your head comfortably on the head restraint. This helps to reduce the risk of whiplash in case of an accident.

● Check that the seat gives support to the lower back. Use a cushion if the seat has no lumbar support.

tips for driving...

● Take any opportunity when the car is stationary to change your position: turn your head from side to side, shrug your shoulders, wriggle around in the seat to get more comfortable.
● Make a conscious effort to relax a tense grip on the steering wheel.
● Breathe rhythmically and deeply to reduce tension.
● Take frequent breaks (at least one an hour) so that you can stand up and walk around to stretch out the body.
● Avoid twisting around as you get in and out of the car.

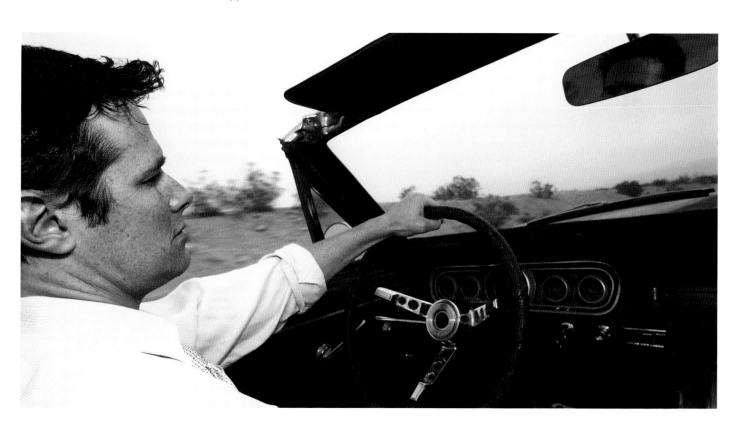

stretches at a desk

If you are working at a desk, stand up and walk around every half-hour or so to stretch out the back. You can also do these simple exercises to relieve any tension. Make sure that your feet are flat on the floor and that you have enough room to stretch.

exercise 1

BELOW Sit well back in your chair. Put the back of one hand in the palm of the other. Raise your arms over your head and bend far enough to the right so that you feel a slight stretch down your left side. Repeat on the other side. Do three stretches on each side.

exercise 2

Interlock your fingers. Slowly raise your arms to chest height. Stretch them away from you, turning your palms outward as you do so. Lower your hands and repeat three times.

safety tip...

Check with a physician before doing these exercises if you have a back problem. Forward bends are not suitable for people with a prolapsed disk.

exercise 3

RIGHT Slowly turn to the left, placing your left hand on the back of the chair and the right one on the outside of your thigh. Hold the position, breathing normally, for a few moments. Then return to the center and repeat on the other side. Stretch both sides again.

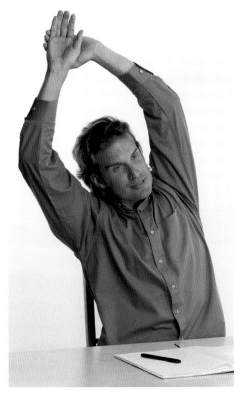

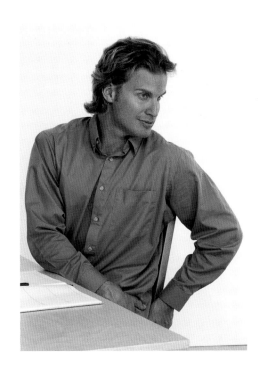

tip...

When you answer the phone, don't cradle it between your shoulder and ear—this strains the neck. Use your hand to hold the receiver, or if you need to use your hands, a headset.

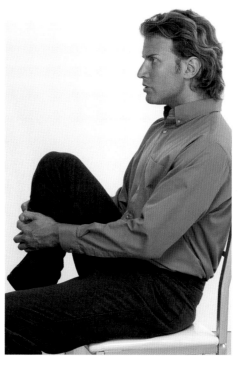
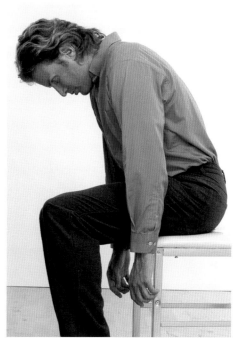

exercise 4

Move your chair away from your desk so you have room to bend forward. Sit on the front of the seat. Contract your abdominal muscles. Slowly lower your chin toward your chest. Then continue the movement down the spine by bending slowly forward. Let your arms hang down. Hold the pose for a few moments, then do the movement in reverse to come up so that you raise the head last. When you are upright, arch the back backward slightly, hold the stretch for a few moments, then return to sitting upright.

exercise 5

ABOVE Cup the right shin just under the knee with both hands. Slowly raise the knee toward your chest and hold the position, breathing normally, for a few moments. Release and do the same on the left leg. Do the exercise once more.

exercise 6

ABOVE Roll forward on your sitting bones so that your bottom sticks out and the arch in your lower back is exaggerated. Then roll backward so that the bottom comes forward and the lower back rounds. Do this rolling movement three times, and finish by finding the midway neutral position between the two extremes.

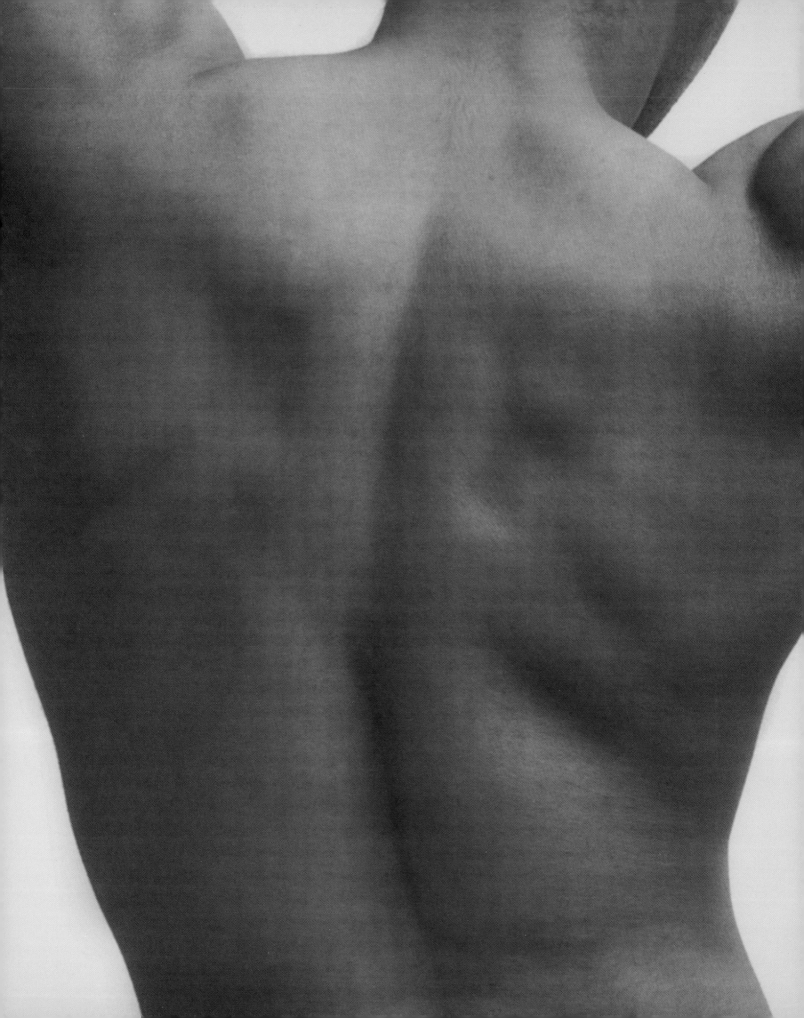

3. waking up your spine

Spending a few minutes each morning doing some simple exercises will help to stretch out your spine after long hours asleep. You can do this routine as soon as you wake up, or at any time during the day—it is good to do after a long period sitting at a desk, for example. You can also use the routine to warm up for the more strenuous back exercises in the following chapter.

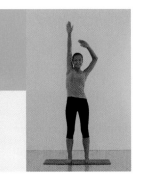

morning stretches

Doing a few gentle movements in the morning will stretch out the spine and help to get your circulation going, sending blood and oxygen to your muscles and ligaments.

stretch up

step 1

Take a few moments to stand and breathe deeply. Stand tall, with your feet hip-width apart, your arms by your sides.

step 2

BELOW LEFT Very slowly, bring your arms up in a wide circle and above your head. Don't exaggerate the movement; let it be natural.

step 3

RIGHT Stretch one arm up, letting the elbow of the other arm bend slightly. Then stretch the other arm up in the same way. Repeat these alternate movements three or four times, as if you are pulling on a rope. Keep your head level, looking straight ahead of you. To end, slowly circle the arms down again.

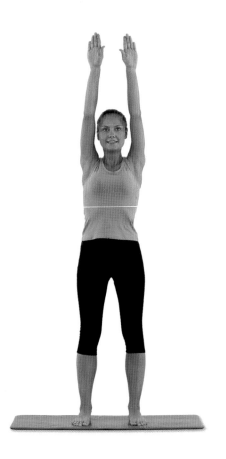

caution...

The stretches in this chapter are suitable for most people. However, they are general exercises, so it is important that you take individual advice on whether they are suitable for you if you have had any back pain or back problems in the past.

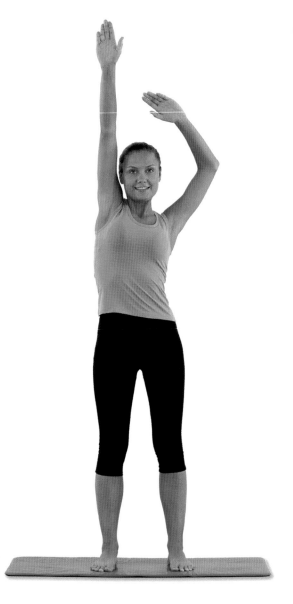

shoulder shrugs

step 1

BELOW Check that your head is held erect and level: pull your chin back and feel your neck lengthen. Then slowly bring your shoulders up toward your ears.

step 3

LEFT Now rotate the shoulders in a clockwise direction 3 or 4 times. Then rotate them in the opposite direction 3 or 4 times.

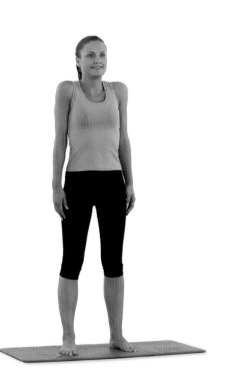

step 2

Let your shoulders slowly drop back down again. Keep your back relaxed as you do this 3 or 4 times.

caution...

Always work slowly and with control, and do not push your body farther than it naturally goes—you should not feel any pain or discomfort when doing these exercises. Over time, you will become more flexible and will naturally be able to stretch farther.

neck stretch

These neck exercises help you to maintain a good range of motion in the neck.
They reduce tension, increase suppleness, and tone the muscles.

step 1

BELOW Tilt your head back so that you can look up. Hold for a few moments, breathing normally, then bring your head back to the front. Slowly drop your chin toward your chest. Again hold for a few moments before bringing back to the central position. Repeat 3 or 4 times.

step 2

LEFT Now turn your head to the right. Hold for a few moments. Return to the central position and repeat on the other side. Repeat.

step 3

Tilt your head to the right, bringing your ear toward your shoulder until you feel a slight pull on the other side of the neck. Keep your head straight as you do so. Hold for a few moments, then return the head to its central position and repeat on the other side. Repeat 3 or 4 times.

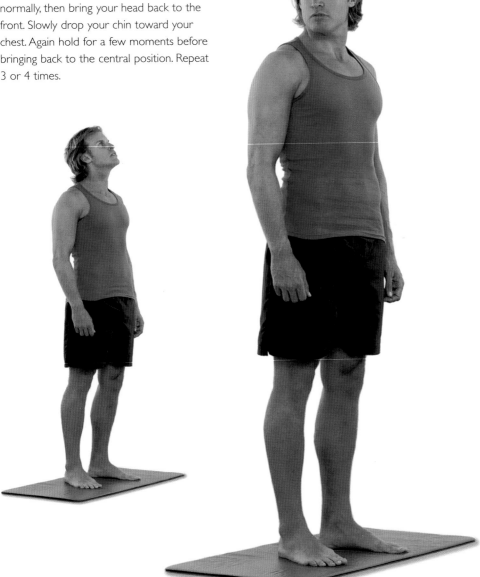

caution...

Don't try to push your neck too far when doing these stretches. See your healthcare provider for advice before doing these exercises if you have a specific neck problem.

chest opening

Opening up the chest helps you to breathe in deeply, using the full capacity of the lungs. This exercise also helps to relax the shoulders.

step 1

BELOW Stand tall with your feet hip-width apart, arms by your sides. Raise your arms to shoulder height, then fold them at the elbows so that your hands are in front of your chest.

step 2

LEFT Open your arms wide to the sides, keeping the elbows slightly bent. Repeat the action 3 or 4 times.

step 3

BELOW Now lower your arms and put your hands behind your back. Interlock your fingers and pull your shoulders back and down. Hold for a few moments, breathing normally and noticing how the chest expands. Repeat 3 or 4 times.

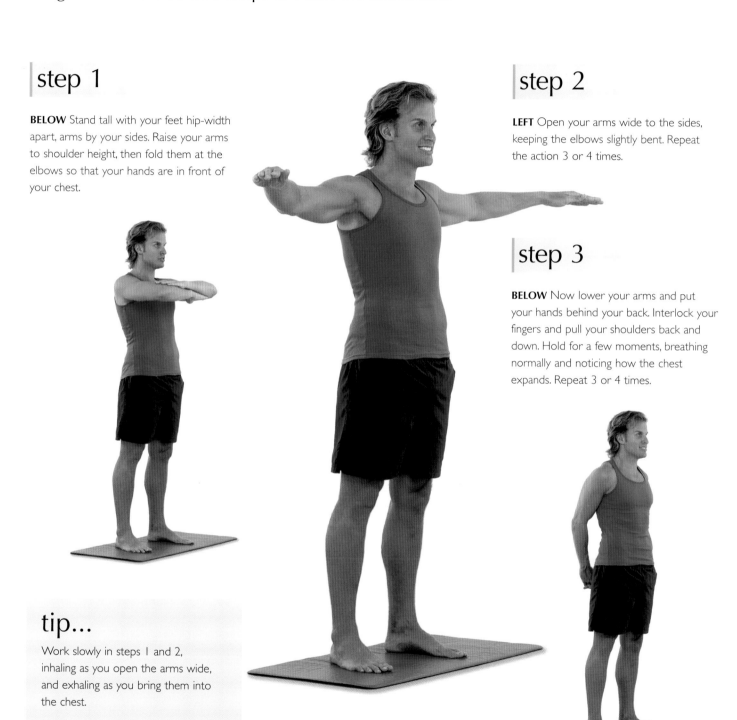

tip...

Work slowly in steps 1 and 2, inhaling as you open the arms wide, and exhaling as you bring them into the chest.

hip shunt

The hip shunt helps to improve suppleness in the lower back as well as the hips. Keep your upper body as still as possible while you do it.

step 1

BELOW Start by standing tall with your arms by your sides, your feet hip-width apart, your hips level, and your knees straight.

step 2

LEFT Slowly bring your weight onto your left leg as you push the left hip outward. Try to keep your shoulders in the same central position as when you were standing upright. Hold for a moment or two, breathing normally.

step 3

Return to the central position, and then bring your weight onto the right leg and push the right hip to the side. Repeat 3 or 4 times, making the movement between left and right smooth and continuous.

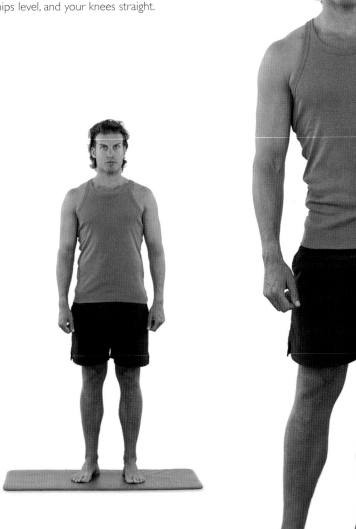

back twists

Gentle back twists from a standing position are easy to control; it is hard to push yourself too far. They give the spine a satisfying stretch, rotating the vertebrae, and working the muscles of the back.

step 1

BELOW Stand tall, with your feet hip-width apart. Put your hands on your hips.

step 2

LEFT Slowly turn to the right as far as you comfortably can. Start the turn from the hips, lifting the spine upward as you turn. Keep the neck and head in line with the spine—don't try to turn the head farther since this will put pressure on the neck. Hold the twist for a few moments, breathing normally.

step 3

Slowly turn back to the center. Then repeat on the other side.

tip...

Try to coordinate your breathing with the movement. Take a deep breath in before you turn, then twist as you breathe out. Return to the center on an out-breath too. This helps you to control the movement.

side bends

These exercises work the muscles at the side of the trunk and help to mobilize the whole spine. You may find it helps to place the opposite hand on your head, but resist any temptation to "push" yourself downward.

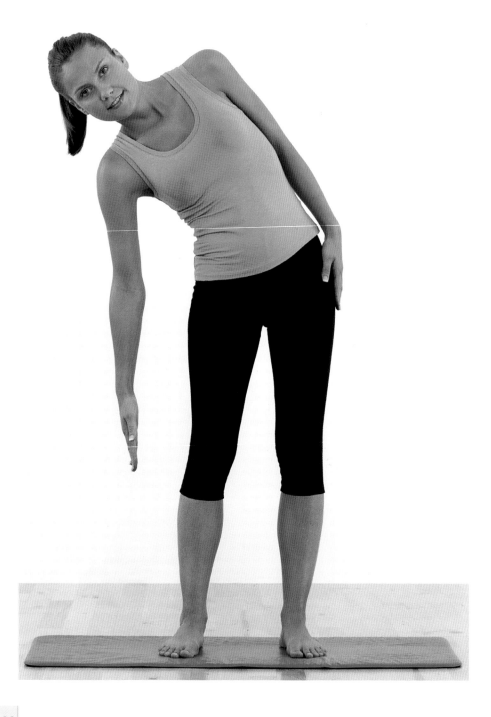

step 1

LEFT Stand tall, with your feet hip-width apart and your arms by your sides. Keeping your pelvis level, bend sideways to the right so that your shoulder comes toward the floor. Let your arm hang down as you bend.

step 2

Stop when you feel a stretch on the opposite side of your waist. Hold for a few moments, and then slowly come up to a standing position. Repeat the stretch 3 or 4 times.

step 3

Now do the same on the other side, stopping as soon as you feel the stretch on your oblique muscles (side of waist). Again, repeat 3 or 4 times.

tip...

Exhale as you bend sideways, then inhale and come up. Exhale in the standing position, inhale, and then bend to the other side as you exhale again.

bending the back

Forward bends help to improve the mobility of the spine, but it is very important that you do them in the correct way: curling from the top of the spine downward and uncurling in the reverse order. Always follow a forward bend with a backward bend.

step 1

Stand tall, with your feet hip-width apart and your arms by your sides. Very slowly bend your head so that your chin drops toward your chest.

step 2

RIGHT Continue bending forward: the head and neck bend first, then the upper back, then the lower back, and then the hips. Do not bend from the waist. Let your arms hang down and remember to keep breathing normally. Hold the pose for 10 seconds or so. Relax.

step 3

Very slowly, reverse the movement so you gradually uncurl to a standing position, bringing the head up last of all.

caution...

Check with your healthcare provider before doing forward bends if you have a back problem. Do not attempt a standing forward bend if you have a prolapsed disk.

step 4

BELOW RIGHT When you are in the upright position, very gently stretch up from the hips and arch backward—you may find this easier if you put your hands on your hips. Hold for a few moments, breathing normally.

step 5

Finally, stand upright and take a few deep breaths to relax completely.

tip...

The back arch is a good exercise to do regularly throughout the day to counteract the effects of slouching.

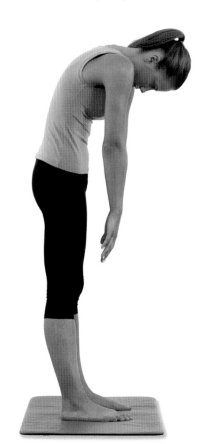

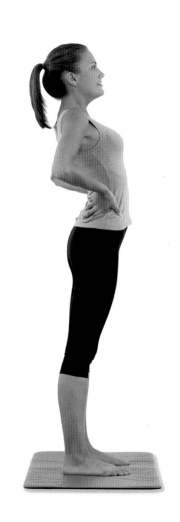

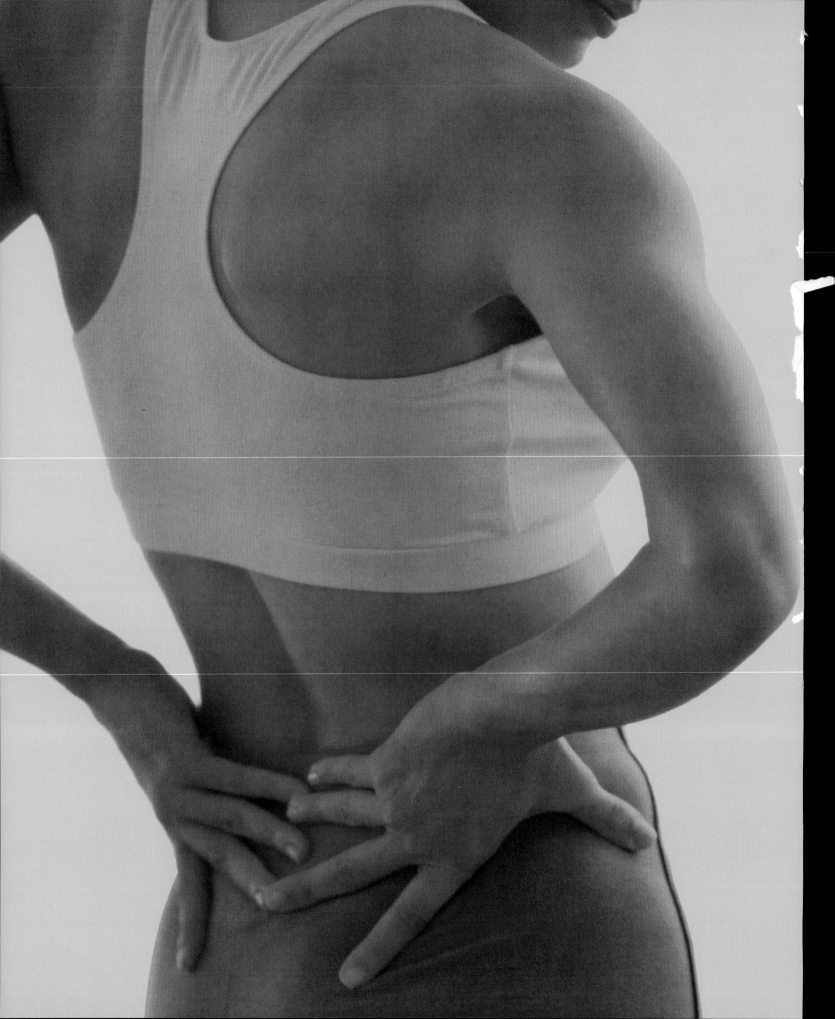

4. mobilizing and strengthening the back

Specific back exercises, such as the ones in this chapter, will help to keep your back healthy. Some are stretches to improve flexibility, others help to increase the tone and strength of your muscles. Warm up before you start, and go only as far as feels comfortable. Back exercises should not hurt: do not try to force your body beyond its capabilities.

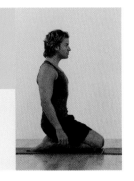

exercising safely at home

You don't need any special equipment to do most back exercises at home. However, you do need a clear space in which to practice, to be dressed sensibly, and work out within your limits.

getting ready

Firstly, clear furniture out of the way. Wear loose comfortable clothing that does not restrict your movements, and have your feet bare. Make sure that you are warm enough—being cold will cause you to tense the muscles. Work on a nonslip surface, such as carpet, or on a special exercise mat. Some exercises can be done using weights, which you can buy from sports stores.

breathing

Do not hold your breath at any point. Keep breathing when you move and when you hold a particular position. Don't speed up a movement to keep up with your breathing; stop and take extra breaths whenever you need to.

slow and steady

Don't try to rush your exercise routine. It is better not to do an exercise at all than to do it in a hurry. Start your routine by spending a few moments standing quietly and taking a few deep breaths to help you relax. When you have stretched as far as is comfortable, hold your position for a few moments, remembering to breathe normally. Over time, this will encourage suppleness in the muscle. Most of the exercises should be repeated several times. Gradually build up the number of repetitions you do; start with three or four repetitions only, building up to ten over time. End your routine with at least five minutes rest, lying on your back. Keep your knees bent and your feet flat on the floor if you feel any pressure in your lower back when you have the legs out straight.

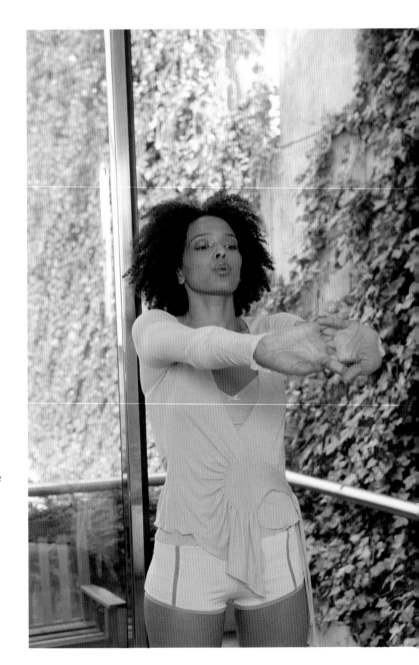

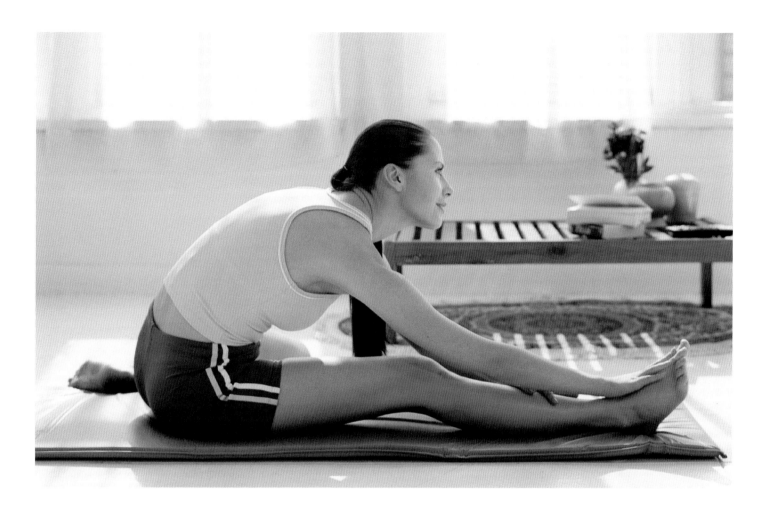

posture

Be conscious of your posture as you exercise. To protect your back, draw up your pelvic floor muscles and then pull in your abdominal muscles. It is also important to keep your hips level and your pelvis in a neutral position rather than tilted. Keep your body in line—not twisted in any way—and relaxed.

safety issues

None of the exercises should cause you any pain. The most you should feel is a gentle stretching sensation. Always respect the limitations of your own body. Stop doing any exercise if you experience pain, and seek medical advice if you are concerned. Do not exercise when you are ill or if you are suffering acute back pain. Back exercises can exacerbate an existing injury or cause

injury if not done correctly. You should always talk to your healthcare provider before beginning a new program of exercise to check that it is suitable for you. This is especially important if you have current or past back problems or other health issues. If you are pregnant, you need to practice special antenatal exercises; the exercises in this book are not suitable.

Before doing any exercise, you should warm up the body by doing some gentle stretches, such as the ones in this chapter, together with some brisk exercise, such as walking on the spot for five minutes. Do the same stretches at the end of your routine to cool the body down.

back press

For back exercises to work, you need to get your pelvis in a level, neutral position. Using a wall helps you to feel your way into neutral. You can practice it at any time during the day.

step 1

RIGHT Stand tall with your back to the wall and your feet a little distance away from it so that you can soften your knees. Keep your head up rather than resting it back against the wall.

step 2

Push your lower back flat against the wall. Hold for a count of five, and then release. Repeat up to ten times.

tip...

Place your feet about 3–4 in (7.5–10 cm) away from the wall so that you can easily flatten your lower back against it. This also helps to make sure that you keep the knees soft rather than locked.

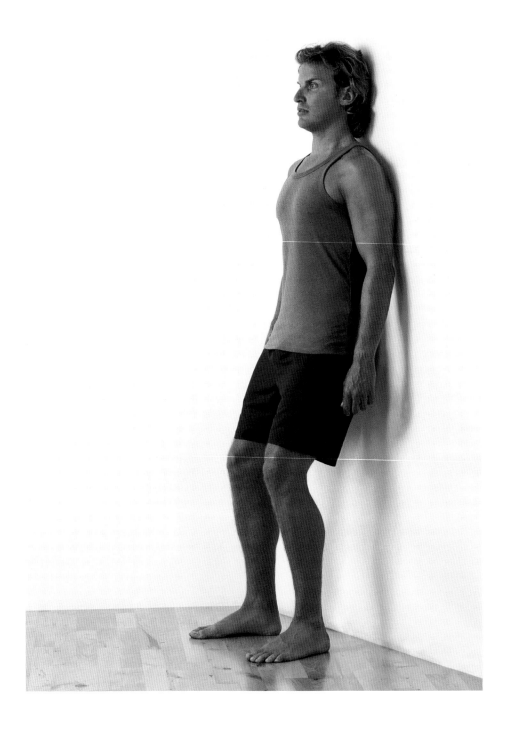

lying-down pelvic tilts

The pelvic tilt will help you to find the neutral position for your pelvis when you are lying down. Repeat the exercise at any point during your routine if you think your pelvis is tilting forward or backward.

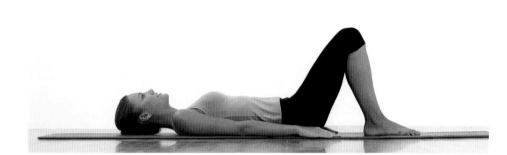

step 1

LEFT Lie on your back with your knees bent, your feet flat on the floor, and your arms by your sides.

tip...

The pelvic tilt provides a gentle stretch for the muscles and ligaments of the back and it also strengthens the abdominal muscle.

step 2

BELOW Press the small of your back into the floor. At the same time, tighten the pelvic and abdominal muscles and squeeze the buttock muscles so that your pelvis tilts upward. If possible, try to get your buttocks to rise a little way off the floor. Hold the stretch for a count of five, then relax. Repeat up to five times.

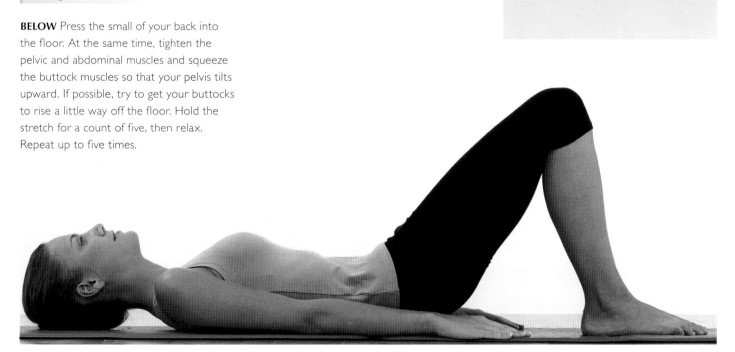

knee hugs

Gentle knee hugs stretch and relax the muscles and ligaments of the lower back and can help relieve aching. Do not do this exercise if you have a prolapsed disk.

step 1

RIGHT Lie on the floor with your knees bent, your feet flat on the floor, and your arms by your sides. Tighten your pelvic and abdominal muscles and push the lower back into the floor.

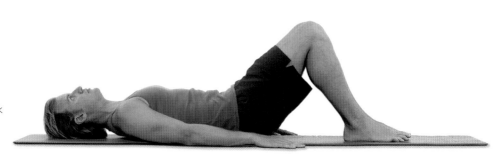

step 2

BELOW Lift your knees up toward your chest, using your hands to pull them toward you. Bring them as close to the chest as you comfortably can. Hold the position for a count of five, breathing all the time.

tip...

This is a good exercise to do if you feel pain in the lower back. Do not raise your head as you do the exercise, or straighten your legs as you bring them back to the floor.

step 3

Gently lower the feet back to the floor one at a time. Repeat up to ten times.

supine twist

This exercise twists the spine, helping to bring the vertebrae into the correct alignment. It stretches the side and lower-back muscles and works on the shoulder and hip joints.

step 1

BELOW Lie on your back with your knees bent, feet flat on the floor, and your arms by your sides.

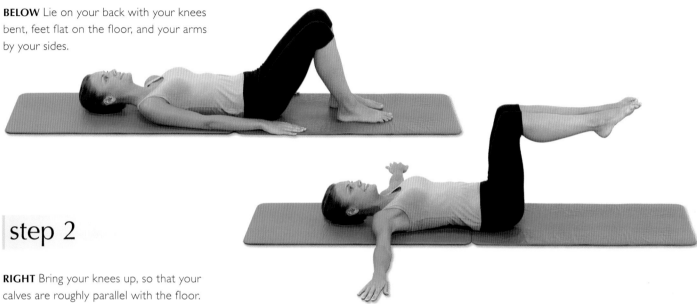

step 2

RIGHT Bring your knees up, so that your calves are roughly parallel with the floor. Open your arms out to the sides. Very slowly, let both knees drop to one side as far as feels comfortable; don't try to force them to the floor. Keep your shoulders and back as flat on the floor as you can. Hold for a count of five, breathing smoothly. Let your legs drop farther toward the floor with each breath. Relax.

step 3

BELOW Bring your legs back to the central position and then drop them over to the other side. Again, hold for a count of five. Repeat up to ten times.

tip...

It is helpful to breathe out as you bring the knees toward the floor, and breathe in as you bring them up.

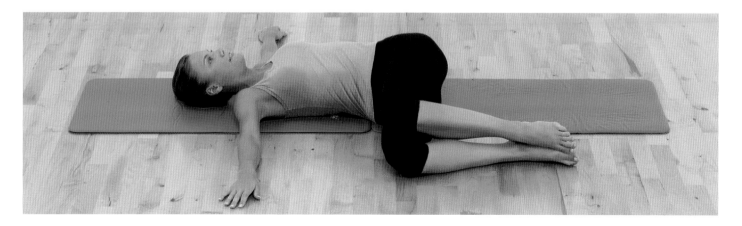

cat pose

This exercise strengthens the back and pelvis and is good for improving the general flexibility of the spine.

step 1

RIGHT Go onto your hands and knees. Your knees should be hip-width apart, feet pointing back. Your wrists should be directly underneath your shoulders, with your fingers spread and facing forward. Keep your arms slightly bent; do not lock the elbows. Look down so that your head, neck, and back are in line.

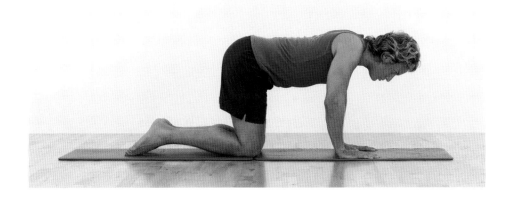

step 2

LEFT Arch your back upwards, dropping your head between your arms as you do so. Hold for a count of five, breathing normally.

step 3

RIGHT Now hollow your back, bringing your head up so that you can look straight ahead. Again, hold for a count of five, breathing normally. Repeat 3 or 4 times.

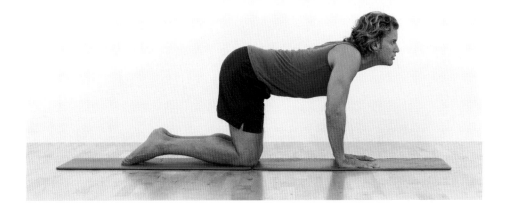

kneeling forward bend

It is good to spend a few moments resting in this forward bend after doing the cat pose. It gives the spine a gentle stretch and is wonderfully relaxing.

step 1

RIGHT From the cat pose, sit back on your calves.

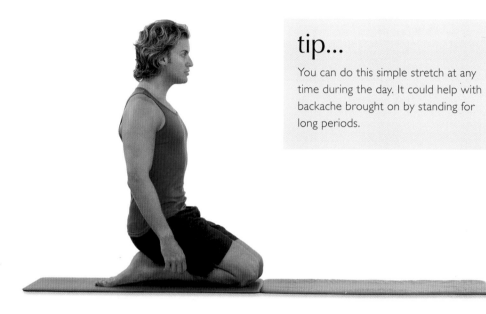

tip...

You can do this simple stretch at any time during the day. It could help with backache brought on by standing for long periods.

step 2

BELOW RIGHT Slowly bend forward, resting your abdomen and chest on your thighs, and letting your forehead rest on the floor in front of you.

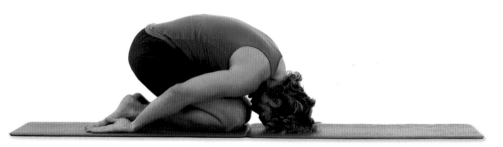

step 3

BELOW Bring your arms forward so you can place your hands and wrists flat on the floor. Hold the position for a minute or two, breathing smoothly. Come up slowly.

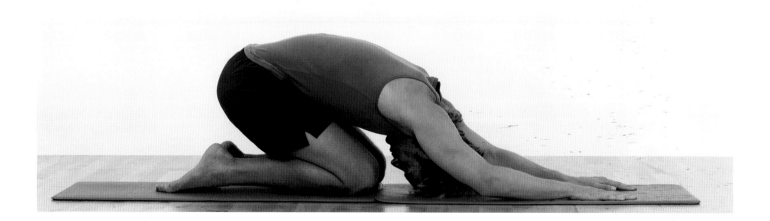

seated twist

Like the supine twist, this exercise helps to improve the back's mobility in turning from side to side. It also feels really good.

step 1

RIGHT Sit upright with your legs out in front of you. Bend your right leg, lift the foot and place it on the mat so that it rests against the outside of your left calf. Rest your left elbow on your right knee and your left hand on your thigh.

tip...

If you find it difficult to keep your back straight when sitting on the floor, try doing a twist while seated on a chair—see page 28.

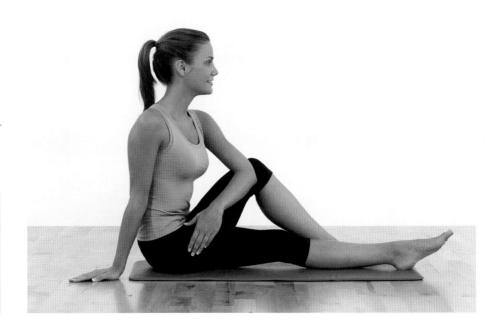

step 2

LEFT Breathe in and extend the spine upward. Breathe out and very slowly turn to the right. Hold for a count of five, breathing normally.

step 3

Breathing out, return to the central position. Then change the position of your legs and arms, and repeat on the other side. Repeat on both sides once more.

back arch

This exercise helps to stretch the spine backward, countering the effects of slouching. Go only as far as feels comfortable.

step 1

RIGHT Lie down on your front. Keep your legs together, tuck your toes under, and place your hands just under your shoulders (as if you were preparing to do a pushup).

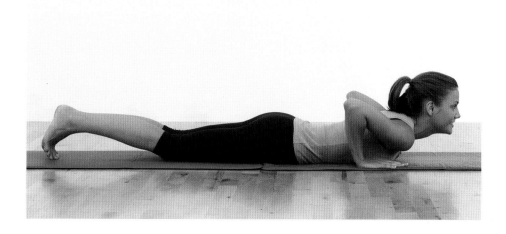

step 2

LEFT Very slowly straighten your arms, lifting your head and shoulders upward. Breathe in as you do so. Hold the position for a count of five, breathing, then slowly lower yourself back down.

step 3

Repeat up to ten times. As you repeat the exercise, you may find that you can go a little farther each time. However, do not try to force your back up.

tip...

Many people find this an excellent exercise for relieving lower-back pain. However, do not do it if it increases your pain. Build up the number of repetitions gradually and raise the back only a little way off the floor at first.

shoulder stretch

This is a good exercise to improve mobility in the upper back, where many people stiffen as they get older. Practiced regularly, it can help to reduce rounded shoulders.

step 1

BELOW Stand in a doorway with your knees bent. Stretch up your arms and grasp the sides of the doorway above your head (your arms should be straight).

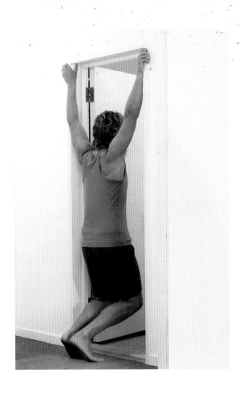

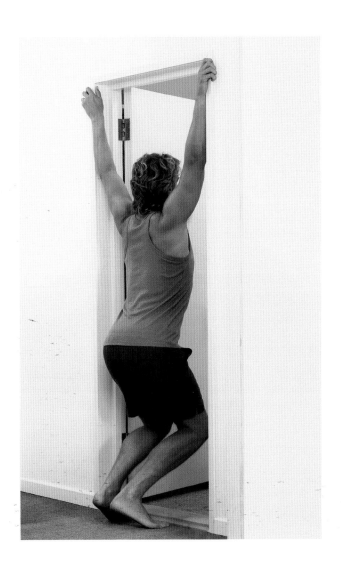

tip...

Keep your elbows straight (but not locked) as you push forward. This is a useful exercise to do if you tend to work at a computer for long periods.

step 2

ABOVE Push forward with your chest (not your stomach) until you feel a stretch in the arms, shoulders, and upper back. Keep your head and neck in line with your spine. Hold the position for a count of five, breathing normally, then relax. Repeat 3 or 4 times.

side stretch

This works the lower back, increasing its flexibility. It needs to be done against a wall. You don't need to go far in order to get a stretch.

step 1

BELOW Stand tall with your back against a wall and your feet slightly away from it so that you can soften your knees slightly. Press your lower back into the wall.

step 2

RIGHT Reach up over your head with your arms, letting them rest against the wall. Then slowly stretch to one side, reaching up with the uppermost arm as you do so. Just go far enough to feel a slight stretch in your lower back and across the pelvis. Hold for a count of five.

step 3

Slowly return to the starting position and do the same on the other side. Repeat up to ten times.

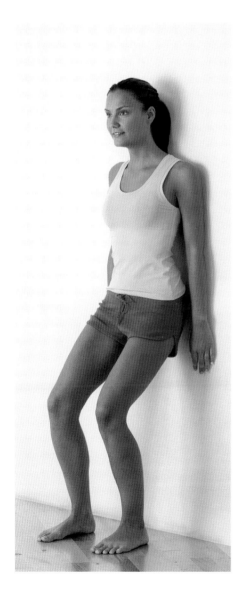

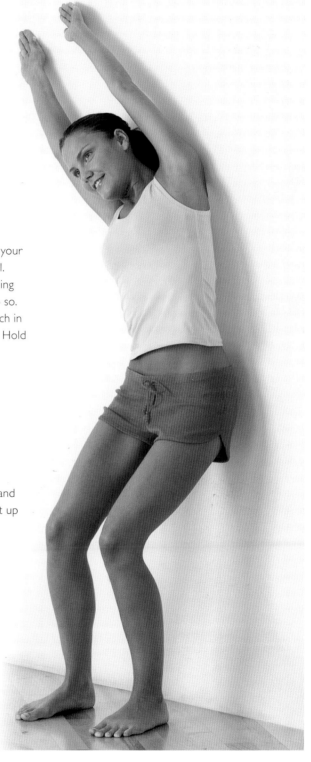

single leg lift

This exercise and the shoulder raise and double leg lift exercise, opposite, help to strengthen the muscles of the back.

step 1

RIGHT Lie on your front, legs together, and arms folded so that you can rest your chin on them.

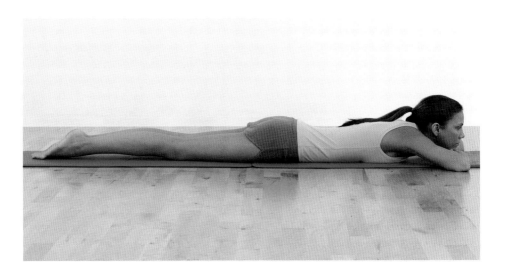

step 2

LEFT Very slowly, raise one leg as you breathe in. Keep it stretching back as you do so, with the toes pointing backward, but do not lock your knee. Lift the leg as far as you can without feeling strain in the back, then hold for a count of five, breathing normally. Bring the leg back down to the floor as you breathe out, and repeat up to ten times.

step 3

Do the same with the other leg, again lifting it only as far as feels comfortable. It doesn't matter if one leg lifts up higher than the other as long as it is comfortable.

tip...

Remember to contract your stomach muscles and to keep your pelvis in a neutral position. Do not arch the back when you lift the leg.

shoulder raise and double leg lift

The shoulder raise and double leg lifts are more difficult than the previous exercise, so you should try them only if you can do single leg lifts easily.

step 1

BELOW Lie on your front, legs together as in the single leg lifts, and rest your head on a towel. This time bring your hands behind your back, placing the back of your left hand in the palm of your right, and rest them on your buttocks.

tip...

Stop straight away if you feel any pain when doing any of these exercises. Do the knee hugs exercise on page 46 to relax the spine.

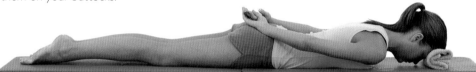

step 2

BELOW Breathe in and bring your shoulders off the ground. Keep looking at the floor, so that your head and neck stay in line with the spine. Hold for a count of five, then breathe out as you lower yourself down to the floor again. Repeat up to ten times.

step 3

BOTTOM OF PAGE Remove the folded towel. Now place your arms by your sides, palms facing upward. Turn your head to one side so that you rest your face on the mat. Then breathe in and raise both legs off the floor simultaneously. Hold for a count of five, then breathe out and return to the floor. Repeat up to ten times.

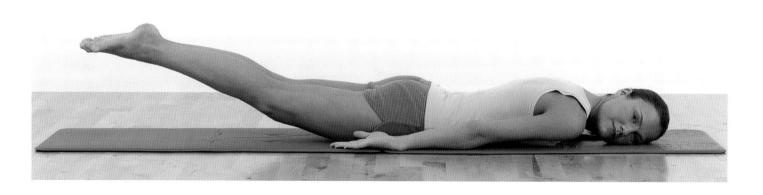

arm raises

You need to keep the spine and pelvis in neutral positions to do this exercise and the following two. They promote core stability, working on the abdominals, buttocks, and legs as well as the back.

step 1

RIGHT Go onto your hands and knees: your wrists should be directly under your shoulders, fingers spread and pointing forward, and your knees should be directly below the hips, toes pointing backward.

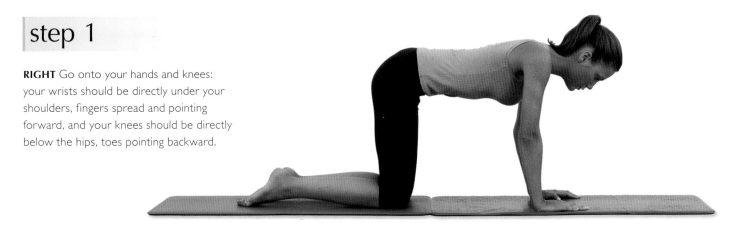

step 2

RIGHT AND BELOW Hollow your back, then arch it. Find the midway neutral point between the positions. Hold for a count of five, breathing normally, to prepare for the arm lifts.

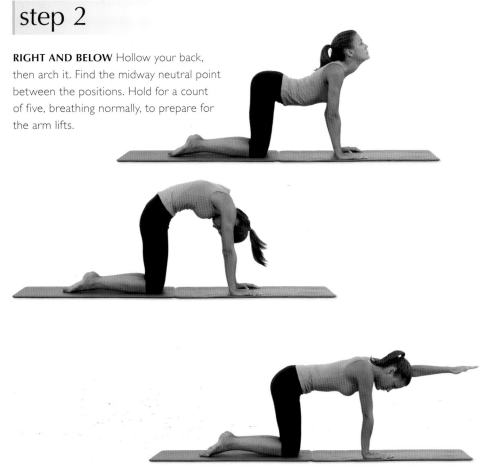

tip...

Remember to keep your pelvic and abdominal muscles pulled in as you do these exercises. Don't raise your arm any higher than horizontal, or you will pull your spine out of alignment. If you find this exercise difficult, start by simply lifting your hand off the floor.

step 3

LEFT Slowly raise one arm until it is parallel with the floor, or as close to horizontal as you can comfortably manage. Keep your head, neck, spine, and pelvis in line. Hold the pose for a count of five, breathing normally, then lower the arm back down to the floor. Repeat ten times, then do the same with the other arm.

leg raises

This exercise is more difficult than the arm raises. Practice it only if you can do the arm raises with ease.

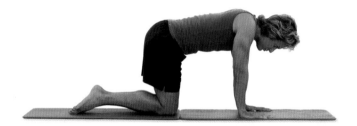

step 1

BELOW Go onto your hands and knees: your wrists should be directly under your shoulders, fingers spread and pointing forward, and your knees should be directly below the hips, toes pointing backward.

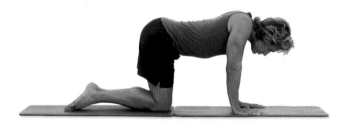

step 2

BELOW Hollow your back, then arch it. Find the midway neutral point between the positions. Hold for a count of five, breathing normally, to prepare for the leg lifts.

step 3

BELOW Now raise one leg until it is parallel with the floor, extending it out behind you. Keep your head, neck, spine, and pelvis in line. Hold for a count of five, breathing normally, then lower the leg back down to the floor. Do ten times, then repeat on the other side.

tip...

Remember to build up the number of repetitions gradually.

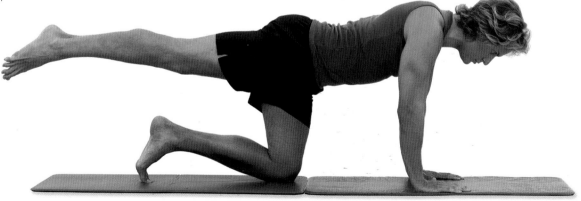

alternate raises

Once you feel completely comfortable with the arm raises and the leg raises, you can try the alternate raises, an exercise that combines the previous two.

step 1

Go onto your hands and knees: your wrists should be directly under your shoulders, fingers spread and pointing forward, and your knees should be directly below the hips, toes pointing backward.

step 2

RIGHT Hollow your back, then arch it. Find the midway neutral point between the positions. Hold for a count of five, breathing normally, to prepare for the arm and leg lifts.

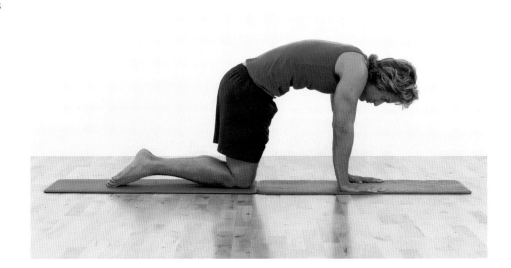

step 3

BELOW Keeping your neck and spine in line and your pelvis in its neutral position, raise the opposite arm and leg simultaneously. Hold for a count of five, breathing normally, then lower the arm and leg back to the floor. Repeat up to ten times and then repeat with the other arm and leg.

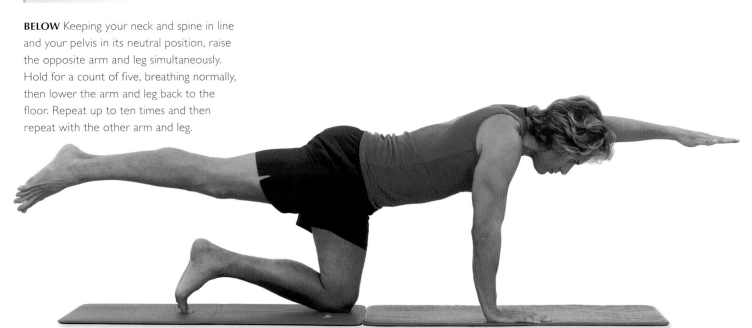

leg lifts

To do this exercise, you need a table that is deep and sturdy enough to support the whole of your torso. This exercise is excellent for working the lower back.

step 1

RIGHT Rest your upper body on the table with your hands holding onto the sides. Make sure that your back is in the neutral position and your pelvic and abdominal muscles are contracted. Slowly raise one leg off the floor until it is in line with your body. Hold the position for a count of five and then return to the floor. Repeat up to ten times, then do the same with the other leg.

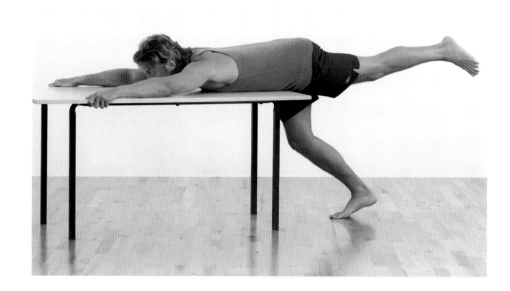

step 2

RIGHT Now lift both legs up simultaneously, raising them until they are level with your body. Hold the position for a count of five, then lower your legs slowly back down to the floor.

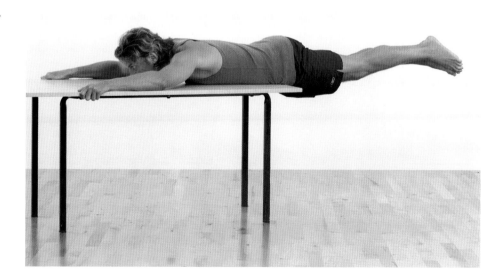

tip...

The double leg lifts in the second step are demanding, so attempt them only when you can do the single leg lifts with ease. Remember to build up the number of repetitions you do gradually.

neck strengthening

These are isometric exercises, meaning that you tense the muscle against a resistant object—in this case, your hand. They are a good way of safely strengthening the muscles of the neck.

step 1

BELOW Press your palm against your forehead and then press against it using the muscles of your neck. Hold for a count of eight and repeat up to ten times.

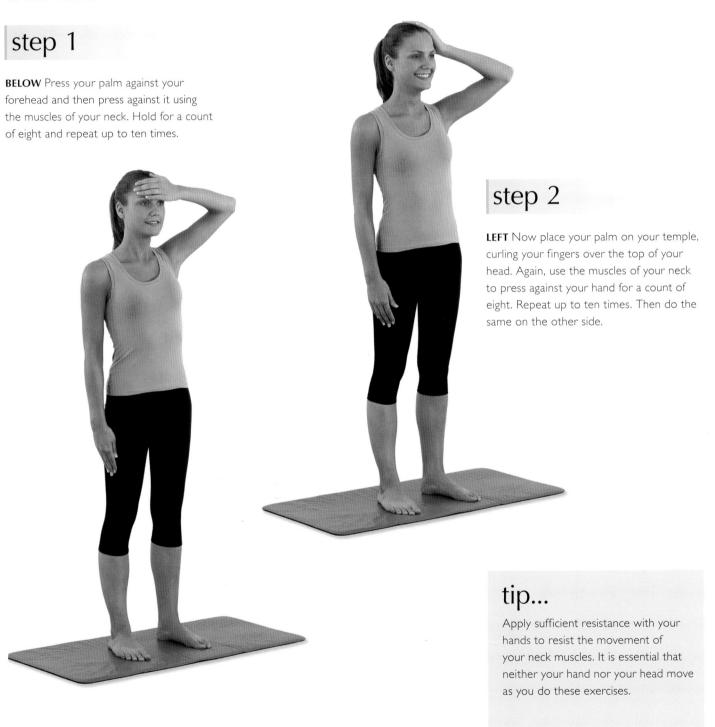

step 2

LEFT Now place your palm on your temple, curling your fingers over the top of your head. Again, use the muscles of your neck to press against your hand for a count of eight. Repeat up to ten times. Then do the same on the other side.

tip...

Apply sufficient resistance with your hands to resist the movement of your neck muscles. It is essential that neither your hand nor your head move as you do these exercises.

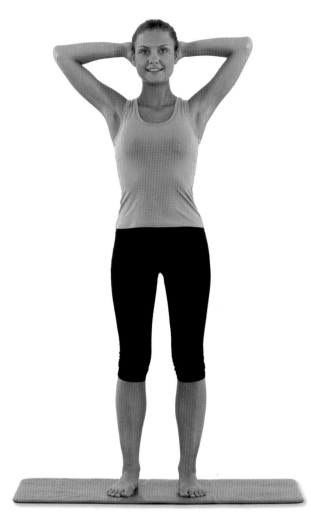

step 4

BELOW Press your right hand over your right temple, letting the fingers curl over the top of your head. Place your left hand on the back of your head so that the heel of your hand is just above your left ear. Now try to turn your head to the right, using your hands to keep your head still. Hold for a count of eight, and repeat up to ten times.

step 5

Then change the position of your hands and do the same on the other side. Again hold for a count of eight and repeat up to ten times.

step 3

ABOVE Place your hands behind your head, interlocking your fingers. Push back into your hands for a count of eight. Repeat up to ten times.

caution...

Don't do these exercises if you can feel stiffness or tension in your neck, as it could exacerbate the problem.

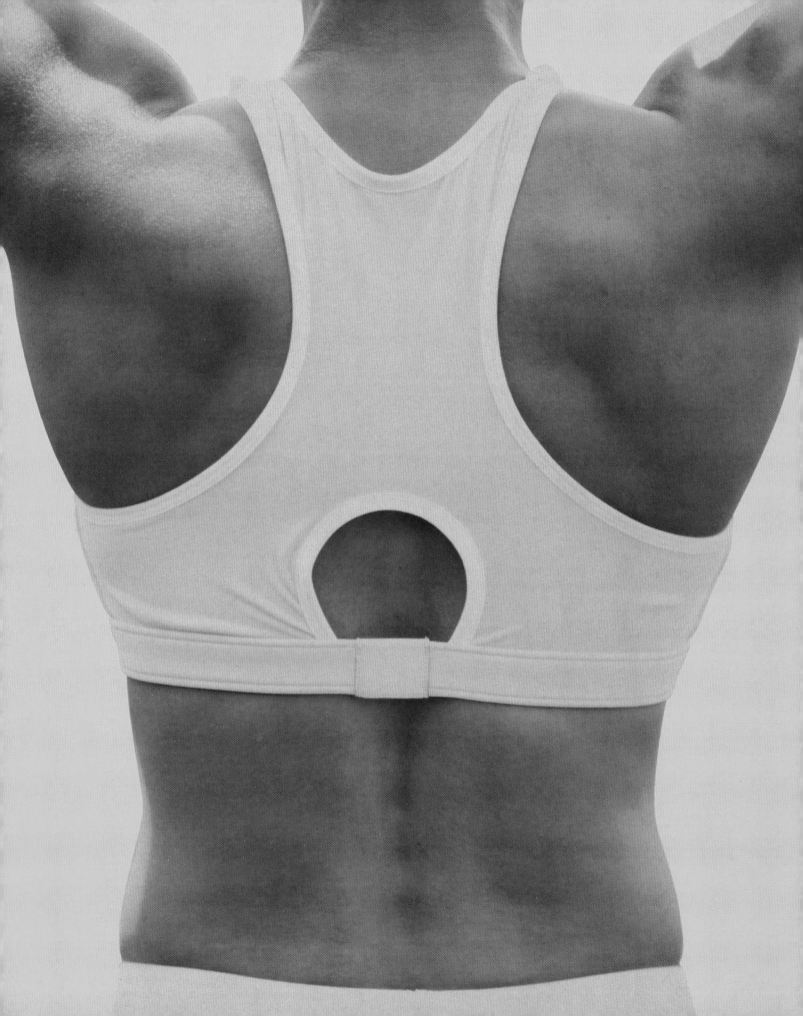

5. abdominals, buttocks, hips, and legs

Any program of exercise for the back should encompass other muscles too. The most important are the abdominals —strong abdominal muscles are essential for developing the core strength that you need to protect your back. But exercising the buttocks, hips, and legs is also an essential part of a complete backcare program.

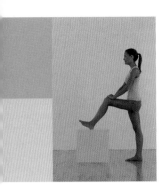

abdominals, buttocks, hips, and legs

Do the following exercises in conjunction with some or all of the back exercises in the previous chapter.

swimming stretch

This exercise works on the abdominals and mimics the movements used during walking. It's good preparation for keeping the lower back still when you are walking in daily life.

step 1

RIGHT Lie on your back, knees bent, feet flat on the floor, and your arms by your sides. Arch your back and then flatten it. Find the midway neutral position between the two extremes.

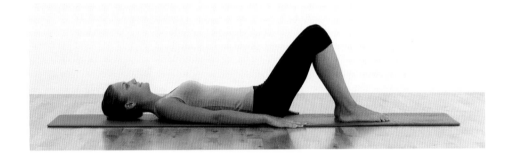

step 2

LEFT Lift your right arm and extend it backward. At the same time, extend your left leg. Hold the position for a count of five, then return your arm and leg to the starting position. Repeat up to ten times.

tip...

Remember to keep your pelvic and abdominal muscles contracted as you do this exercise.

step 3

Now do the same on the other side, extending your left arm and your right leg. Again hold the position for a count of five, then return to the starting position.

oblique press

This is an isometric exercise in which you push against your knee in order to tone the abdominals. It involves a slight turn so it helps the muscles at the sides of the trunk.

step 1

BELOW Lie on your back, knees bent, and feet flat on the floor. Place your arms by your sides. Press your lower back into the floor.

tip...

Keep your back flat on the floor as you do this exercise.

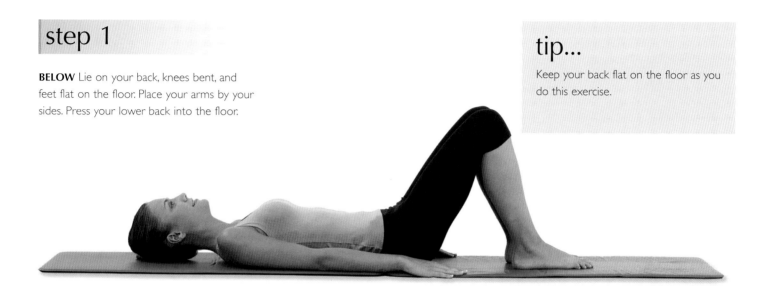

step 2

BELOW Raise your right leg from the floor so that your thigh is at a 90° angle to the floor and your calf is parallel to it. Place the palm of your left hand on your right knee and push against it, resisting the force with your knee so that neither arm nor leg moves position. Hold the position for a count of eight, then relax.

step 3

Do the same with the other leg and hand, again holding the position for a count of eight. Repeat up to ten times on each side.

caution...

Do not do this exercise if you have lower-back pain.

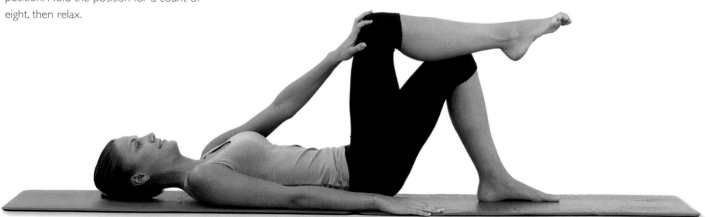

curl-ups

In this exercise you keep the abdominals still while raising the upper body off the floor. It's easier to do than the oblique curl-up, so you should master this first.

step 1

RIGHT Lie on the floor with your knees bent and your feet flat on the floor. Place your arms by your sides and press your lower back into the floor.

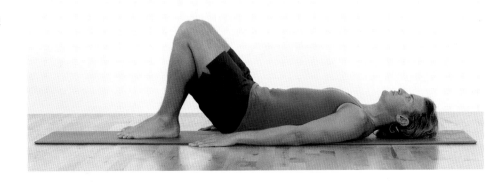

caution...

Do not do curl-ups or oblique curl-ups if you have a neck problem.

step 2

BELOW Slowly raise your head and shoulders off the floor, bringing your chin toward your chest. Reach your arms toward your calves as you do so. Hold the position for a count of five, then very slowly lower the back down to the floor again. Repeat up to ten times.

tip...

As you release the posture, bring the back onto the floor first, followed by the shoulders and then the neck.

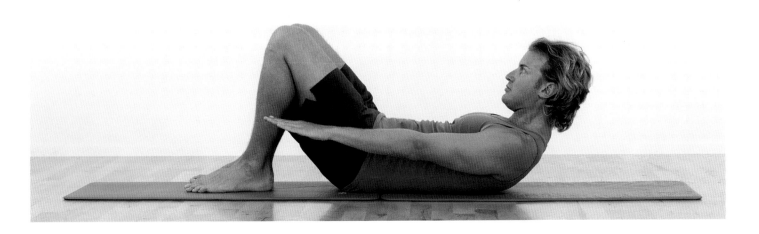

oblique curl-ups

This is an excellent exercise for working the sides of the trunk; it also helps to give the hip flexors a good stretch.

step 1

RIGHT Lie on the floor with your knees bent and your feet flat on the floor. Place your arms at right angles to your body.

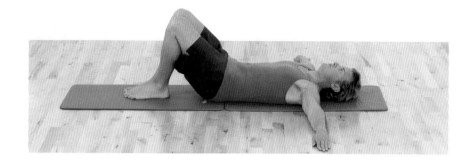

step 2

RIGHT Press your lower back into the floor and bring your knees off the floor so that your lower legs are parallel to the floor.

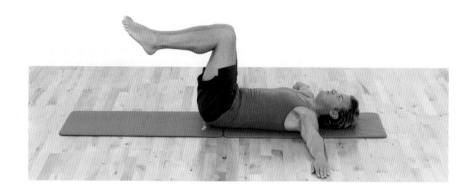

step 3

LEFT Bring your hands to the sides of your head. Then, raising your head and shoulders, bring one elbow toward the opposite knee, bringing the knee back toward the elbow simultaneously. Keep your neck in line with the spine, do not pull on it with your hands.

step 4

Release and repeat on the other side. Repeat the whole exercise up to ten times, working rhythmically and breathing normally throughout. Do not hold the stretch.

buttock stretch

The muscles of the buttocks (gluteals) get a good stretch in this exercise. The deepest gluteal muscle is the piriformis, which plays an important part in stabilizing the pelvis.

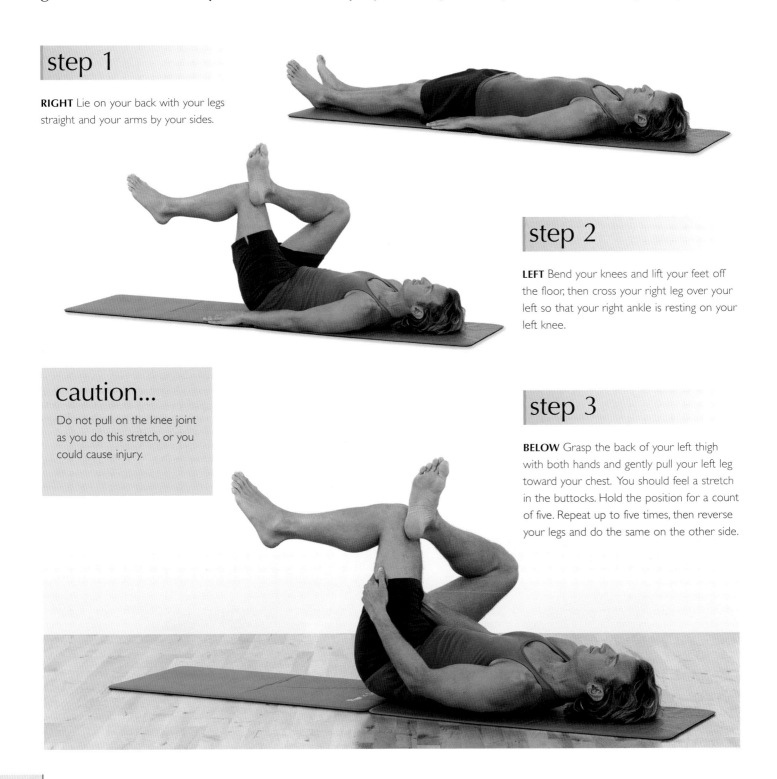

step 1

RIGHT Lie on your back with your legs straight and your arms by your sides.

step 2

LEFT Bend your knees and lift your feet off the floor, then cross your right leg over your left so that your right ankle is resting on your left knee.

caution...

Do not pull on the knee joint as you do this stretch, or you could cause injury.

step 3

BELOW Grasp the back of your left thigh with both hands and gently pull your left leg toward your chest. You should feel a stretch in the buttocks. Hold the position for a count of five. Repeat up to five times, then reverse your legs and do the same on the other side.

hip flexor stretch

If you spend a lot of time sitting down, then your hip flexors (psoas muscles) are likely to shorten. This can pull the pelvis forward and out of alignment.

step 1

RIGHT Kneel on your right knee with your left leg bent in front of you. The right calf and top of the right foot should be resting on the floor and pointing backward. The left thigh should be parallel to the floor and the left foot should be flat on the floor, toes pointing forward. Rest your hands lightly on your left thigh, just above the knee.

step 2

BELOW RIGHT Lean forward, keeping your back and neck in line, and bring your weight onto the left foot. You should feel a stretch in the groin of the right leg. Hold the stretch for a count of five and then release. Repeat on the other side.

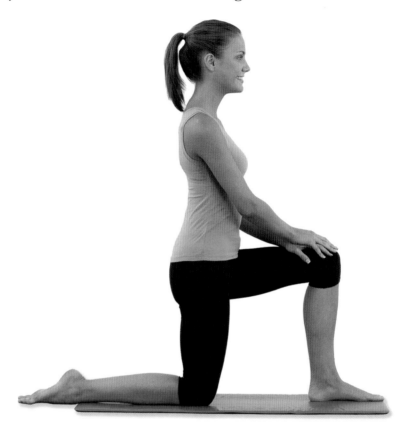

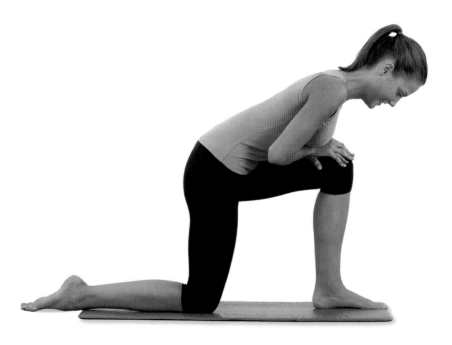

standing hamstring stretch

Many people have tight hamstrings, which can contribute to lower back pain and help to pull the pelvis out of the neutral position.

step 1

BELOW Stand with your right foot flat on the floor and the heel of your left foot on the seat of a chair. Rest both hands on your left thigh, just above the knee.

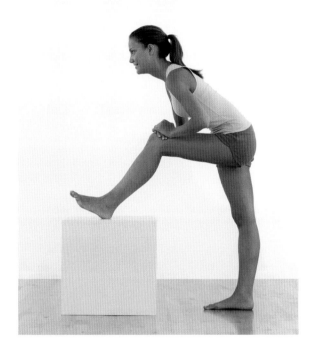

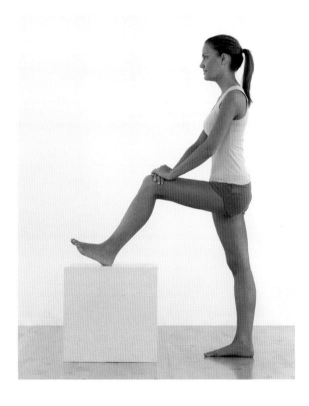

step 2

ABOVE Keeping your back straight, bend from the hips until you feel a slight stretch in the back of the right thigh. Hold the position for a count of five and then release. Repeat up to ten times, then switch legs and do the same on the left side.

caution...

The hamstring stretches may not be suitable if you suffer from sciatica—check with your healthcare provider. You should not feel pain in the lower back when you do these exercises—if you do, seek advice from an expert.

step 3

Once you find that this hamstring stretch becomes easier, increase the challenge by placing your heel against a wall rather than on a chair.

lying-down hamstring stretch

The lying-down stretch is easier to do than the standing one. You will need a resistance band or a scarf to do this exercise.

step 1

RIGHT Lie on the floor with your legs bent and feet flat on the floor. Place your arms by your sides and check that your pelvis is in the neutral position.

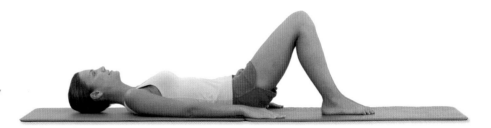

step 2

LEFT Raise one knee toward your chest and place the band around the sole of the foot. Hold one end of the band in each hand.

step 3

BELOW Slowly straighten your leg, pressing through the heel. Hold the position for a count of five and release the tension by bending the leg again. Repeat up to ten times and then do the same on the other leg.

tip...

Straighten your leg enough to feel a stretch on the back of the thigh. Do not force the movement. You can use a scarf instead of a resistance band for this exercise.

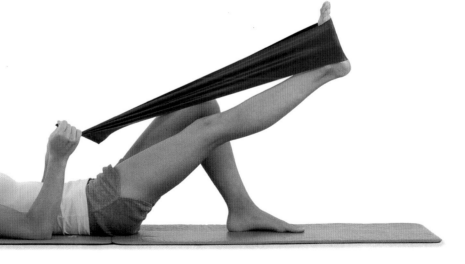

standing calf stretch

Calf stretches help to lengthen the Achilles tendon at the back of the ankle as well as the calf muscles.

step 1

Stand in front of a wall. Put your hands against the wall at shoulder-level.

step 2

RIGHT Take a step back with one foot and place your foot so that it is facing the wall and the heel is on the floor. Slowly lean toward the wall, keeping your back straight, until you feel a stretch in your calf. Hold the stretch for a count of ten, then release. Repeat up to ten times and then change legs and exercise the other side.

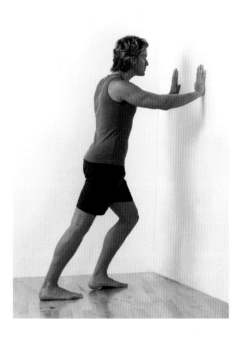

sitting calf stretch

step 1

BELOW Sit with one leg stretched out in front of you and the other bent with the foot flat on the floor. Place a resistance band or scarf around the foot of the straight leg and hold one end in each hand.

step 2

BELOW Slowly raise your leg a little way off the floor, toes pointing directly upward, until you feel a stretch. Hold for a count of five and then release. Repeat up to ten times, then do the same on the other leg.

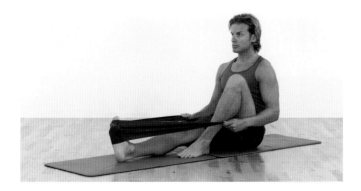

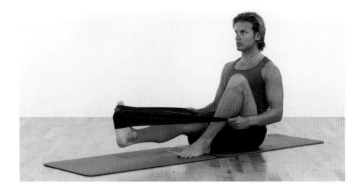

standing quad stretch

The quadriceps are a large muscle group at the front of your thigh, which flexes the hip and extends the knee.

step 1

Stand with the legs together, in front of a wall or a sturdy chair that you can put your hand on for balance. Bend the leg that is farthest away from the wall and grasp the ankle with your hand.

step 2

RIGHT Lift your foot toward the buttocks. Be sure to keep your pelvis in the level, neutral position and to pull the leg up without twisting it. Hold the stretch for a count of five, breathing normally, then release. Repeat up to ten times and then reverse your position and do the same on the opposite leg.

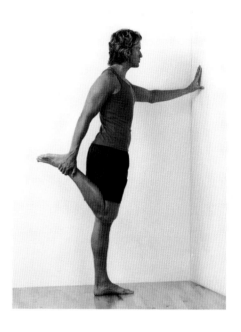

lying-down quad stretch

step 1

RIGHT Lie on your side, bending your elbow so you rest your head in your hand. Bend your uppermost leg behind you and grasp it with your uppermost hand. Bend your lower leg in front of your body if it feels uncomfortable.

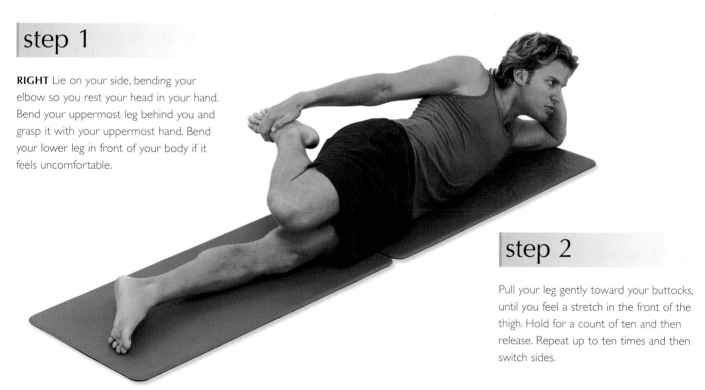

step 2

Pull your leg gently toward your buttocks, until you feel a stretch in the front of the thigh. Hold for a count of ten and then release. Repeat up to ten times and then switch sides.

squats

These are strengthening exercises that work your buttock muscles as well as the quads, hamstrings, and calves. They are quite demanding, so start with just a few repetitions.

step 1

BELOW Stand with your feet hip-width apart, feet facing forward or slightly outward. Make sure that your pelvis is in the neutral position.

step 2

LEFT Slowly bend your knees and lower your buttocks as if you were lowering yourself onto a chair. Keep your pelvic and abdominal muscles pulled in and your spine straight as you do so: don't lean forward. Hold the squat for a count of five, then come up slowly. Repeat up to ten times.

variation...

If you find it hard to keep your back straight, try doing the exercise against a wall. Place your feet far enough away so that you can bend your knees to a 90° angle as you squat. Rest your lower back, shoulders, and head against the wall, and lower yourself into a squat. Again, hold for a count of five and repeat up to ten times.

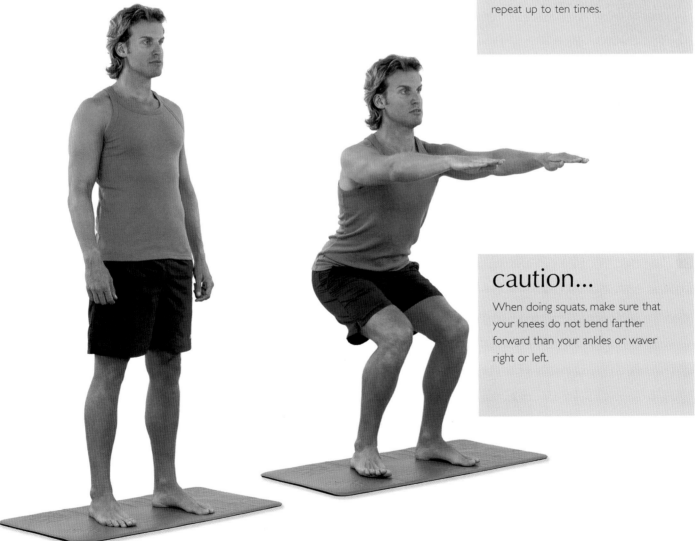

caution...

When doing squats, make sure that your knees do not bend farther forward than your ankles or waver right or left.

lunges

The lunge is a good strengthening exercise that stretches your hip flexors, and also works on most of the muscles of the buttocks and legs as well as the back.

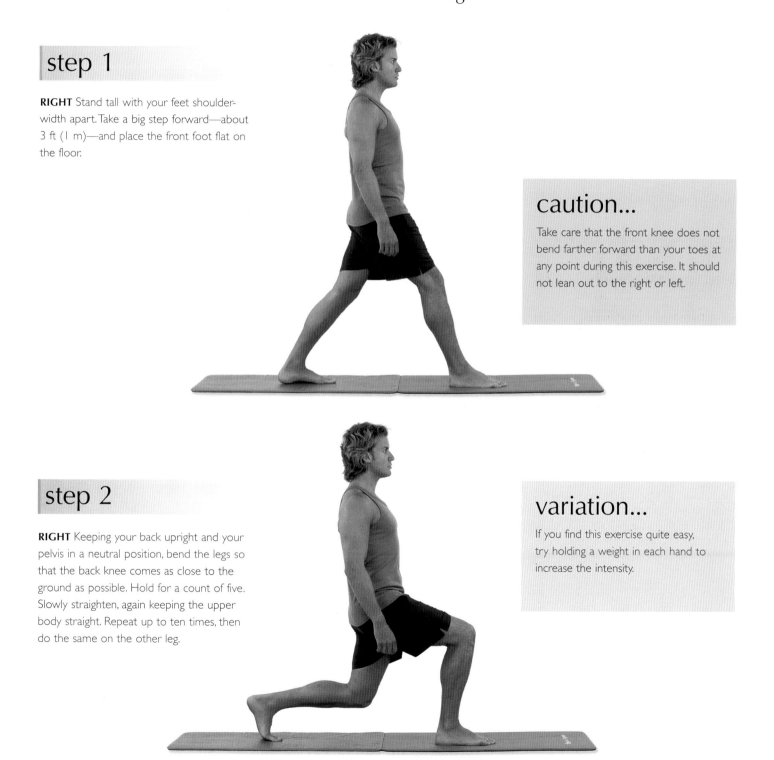

step 1

RIGHT Stand tall with your feet shoulder-width apart. Take a big step forward—about 3 ft (1 m)—and place the front foot flat on the floor.

caution...

Take care that the front knee does not bend farther forward than your toes at any point during this exercise. It should not lean out to the right or left.

step 2

RIGHT Keeping your back upright and your pelvis in a neutral position, bend the legs so that the back knee comes as close to the ground as possible. Hold for a count of five. Slowly straighten, again keeping the upper body straight. Repeat up to ten times, then do the same on the other leg.

variation...

If you find this exercise quite easy, try holding a weight in each hand to increase the intensity.

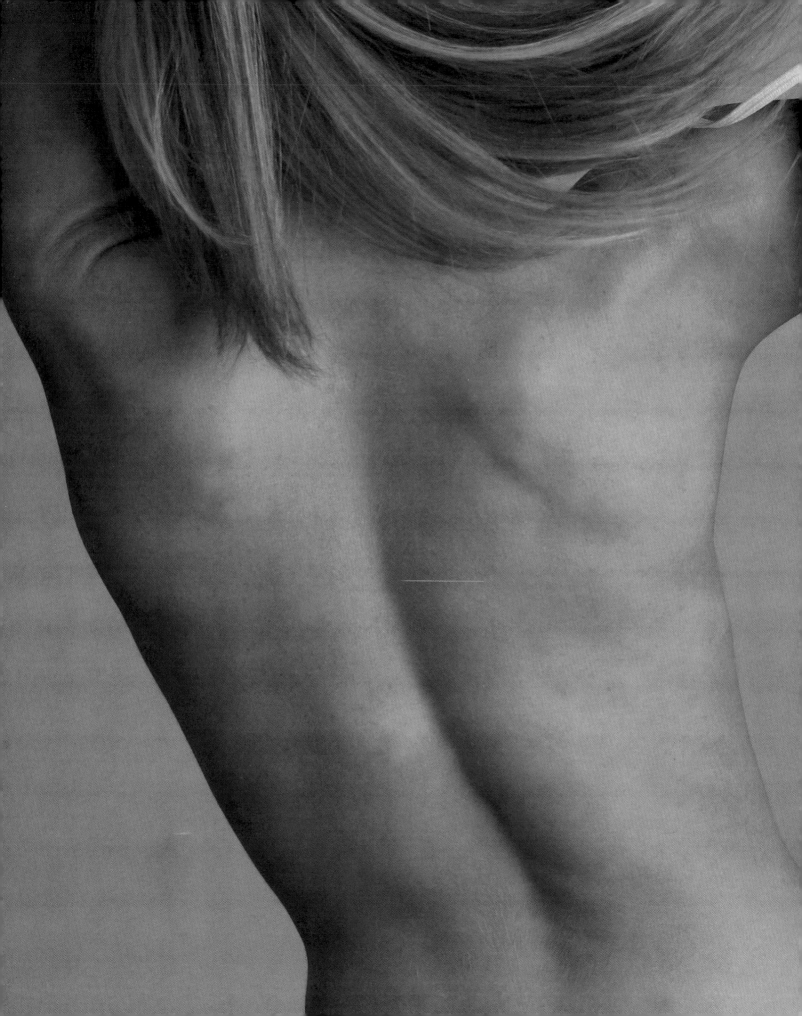

6. understanding back pain

Almost everyone gets back pain at some stage in their lives,
and many people have recurrent back problems.
This chapter gives an overview of the most common causes
of back pain and suggests ways to deal with them.
The lower back, which takes most of the body's weight, is
the most usual place to experience back pain—about six
out of ten people suffer lower-back pain in any given year.

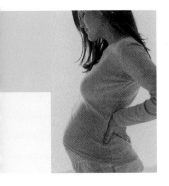

general back pain

Back pain can develop gradually over time or come on very suddenly. It can take the form of a dull ache or a sharp pain, and may restrict movement. But, however severe it may feel, most back pain gets better without treatment.

Most lower-back pain is difficult to diagnose—in 85 percent of cases, the person recovers without the exact cause being determined. But these are some of the likely causes.

muscle strain

It is quite difficult to strain the muscles of the back. But overstretching and tearing can occur after a sudden vigorous movement is performed—for example, when you lift something too heavy for you, or if you undertake strenuous sport without warming up first. The pain comes on suddenly and there may also be swelling and bruising. However, muscles tend to heal rapidly and respond well to rest and physiotherapy.

muscular tension

A more common cause for back pain is muscle tension. It is usually connected to poor posture, which puts the muscles under pressure. For example, leaning over a low table for a long period will strain the muscles of the lower back. Older men who do heavy work are prone to muscle tension, especially if they are overweight.

stretched ligaments

Ligaments are not very flexible, so they can easily become overstretched. They can be damaged in the same way as a muscle, but take longer to heal. The pain is often worse first thing in the morning, or after prolonged sitting or standing. Sufferers often find that they have to change position repeatedly to get comfortable.

lower-back pain in pregnancy

Pregnant women often experience lower-back pain. This is because the growing weight of the baby causes them to lean back as they stand. This puts the muscles and ligaments under pressure. Back pain usually improves after the baby is born. Osteopathy or chiropractic may help to reduce postural strain during pregnancy.

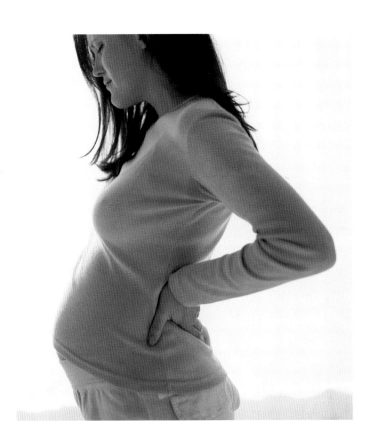

general neck and shoulder pain

After the lower back, the neck and shoulders are the most likely site for pain to occur. Again, muscle tension is a likely cause. For example, if you hold a phone between your ear and your shoulder for a long period, the neck muscles are likely to become tense and achy. Similarly, the shoulder muscles will be placed under pressure if you perform repetitive movements or hold yourself in an awkward position for long periods.

Certain points in the neck and shoulder can then go into spasm and form painful knots. Massage, physiotherapy, or gentle stretching exercises can help to release tension from these "trigger points."

Stress can be a factor in neck pain, since anxiety often leads to a tensing of the muscles here. Massage can relieve stress, as can acupuncture and gentle forms of exercise such as swimming, yoga, or Pilates.

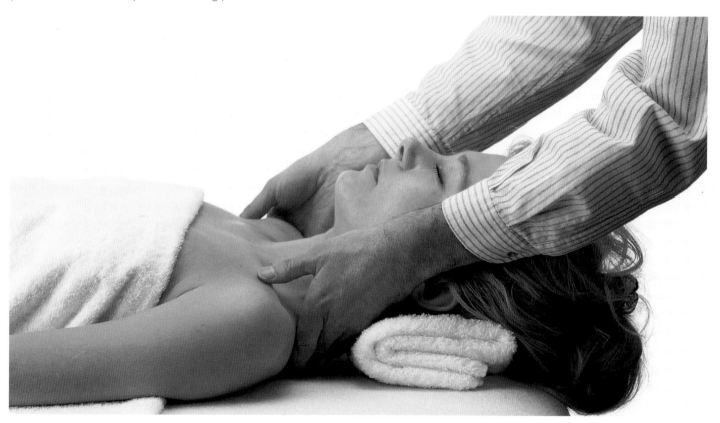

wryneck

Wryneck is a condition where the neck is painful and cannot be turned to one side. The cause is not clear, though it is possible that it is the result of a nerve being pinched between two vertebrae. It usually clears up within a few days, and acupuncture, chiropractic, or osteopathy may help to prevent recurrence.

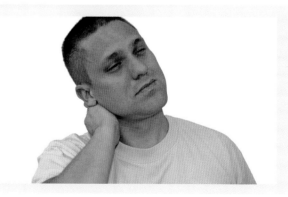

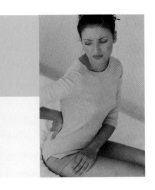

chronic and recurring back pain

Most nonspecific back pain lasts less than two weeks. When pain persists for much longer—12 weeks or more—it is termed chronic.

prolapsed disk

People often talk about having a "slipped disk," but in fact the intervertebral disks cannot slip. But they can burst: the disk may rupture—usually after a sudden twisting movement—causing the jelly-like nucleus to leak out. This can press on the adjacent nerve, causing severe pain that can radiate out into the buttocks, hips, or legs, or into the arm and hand if a disk in the neck is affected. Movement is often restricted and sensation may be lost in certain areas. A physician should be able to pinpoint which nerve is affected from the site of any weakness or numbness. Rest and painkillers can help to relieve the initial pain. But it is important to keep as mobile as possible after the first couple of days, since this hastens recovery.

sciatica

This is pain emanating from the sciatic nerve, which runs down the leg. The most common cause is a prolapsed disk in the lower back, but it can also be due to degenerative changes to the vertebrae and some rarer causes, so you should seek advice from a physician. An attack of sciatica usually starts with lower-back pain, but then shifts to the buttock and leg. You may also experience tingling or weakness in these areas. The pain can be intense but usually eases off after a week or two, although the problem often recurs.

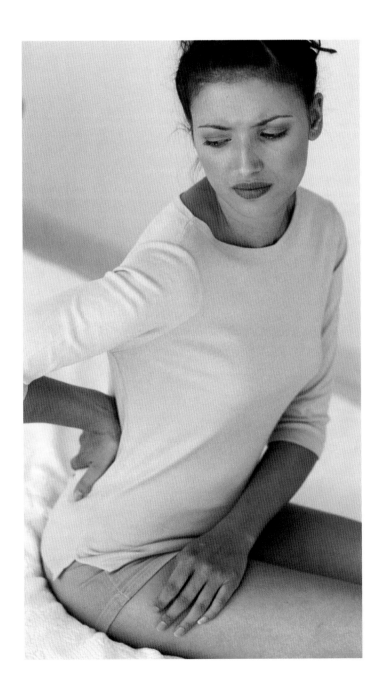

facet joint problems

The facet joints that connect the vertebrae can be damaged by a sudden twisting movement or by conditions such as osteoarthritis. If the joint becomes inflamed, it might press painfully on surrounding tissues, causing pain that can radiate outward to the buttock or thighs. There is no numbness or weakness as in a prolapsed disk. Rest, painkillers, exercises, and manipulation can all be helpful.

disorders affecting the spine

Chronic or recurring pain can also be the result of normal wear and tear, or diseases such as osteoporosis and, very occasionally, cancer. Sometimes pain can be "referred" from another site altogether, so back pain may be due to disease in one of the internal organs such as the kidneys or stomach. It is therefore important that you seek medical advice and get a proper diagnosis if back pain persists.

fractured vertebrae

The vertebrae can fracture if they are subjected to a powerful impact, such as a heavy blow, bad fall, or traffic accident. A minor fracture will cause pain but no long-lasting damage, but in some cases the spinal cord can be affected, which might in extreme cases lead to paralysis or death. If you suspect a fracture, it is essential that you keep still while the emergency services are called.

whiplash

If the neck is jerked violently—as in a traffic accident when the car is hit from behind—then damage is likely to occur. The facet joints, disks, muscles, and ligaments of the neck can all be affected. Symptoms may not occur immediately, but the neck will become very stiff and painful within a day or two. The sooner treatment starts the better, so you should see a doctor if there is any possibility that you have sustained a whiplash injury. Painkillers and exercises to maintain the neck's range of motion are usually helpful, and osteopathy and chiropractic can help.

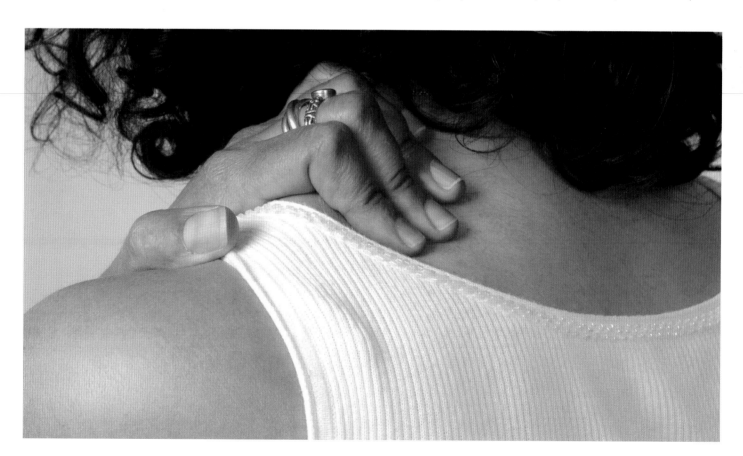

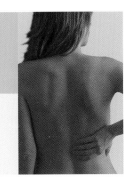

what to do

It is not necessary to see a physician for most cases of simple back pain. A physician is unlikely to be able to diagnose the exact problem and home treatment is usually effective.

when to seek help...

- Keep still and get someone to call the emergency services if there is a possibility of a fracture to the vertebrae—for example, if you have had a bad fall, suffered a heavy blow to the back, or been involved in an accident.

- Go to the emergency department if you are in a car that has been hit from behind or your neck has been violently jolted in another way.

- Get immediate medical advice (by calling your physician or going to the emergency department) if you experience numbness in one or both legs or arms, you are having difficulty passing water or moving your bowels, or you have chest pain as well as back pain.

- See your physician if back pain does not improve after 24 hours with home treatment; the pain is worse on lying down; you have weakness or tingling in the arm or leg; you are over 50 or under 20 years of age; you are pregnant; or you have any other unusual symptoms.

- Revisit your physician if symptoms persist or a chronic condition gets worse.

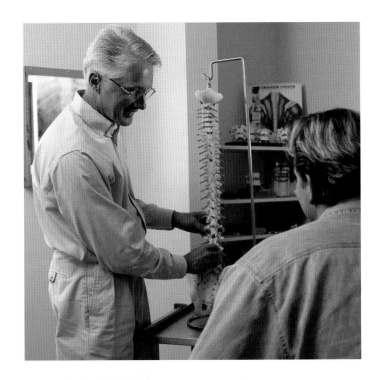

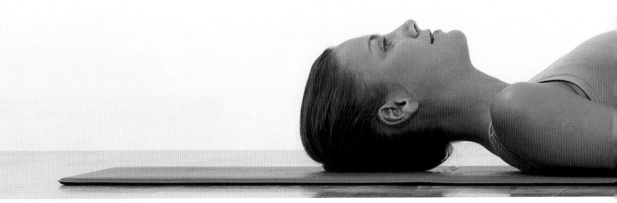

home treatment for back pain

When acute back pain strikes, the best thing to do is to lie down. If possible, lie on a bed; otherwise, lie on the floor (see next page for good positions). People with bad backs used to be advised to go to bed until they felt better. However, it is best to keep as mobile as possible to maintain the back's range of movement, so don't go to bed for longer than a day or two.

Over-the-counter painkillers such as ibuprofen or paracetamol may be enough to manage any pain. Your physician can prescribe something stronger if these drugs are not sufficient.

Applying heat or cold, or a combination of both, can also give temporary pain relief. A hot shower or a hot-water bottle wrapped in a towel can help to soothe muscle strain, while a cold compress or ice pack (left in place for a maximum of ten minutes at a time) can reduce inflammation. Experiment to see which helps your pain most—or try using both: hold a hot-water bottle against the area for a minute, then a cold compress, and keep alternating the two for 15–20 minutes. Gentle massage can be helpful, so long as it is done very gently.

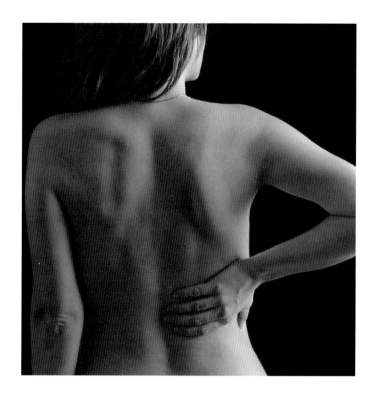

Once the pain starts to ease, continue with normal activities as much as possible. Be aware of your posture and avoid lifting, straining, or sitting or standing for long periods. Back exercises can be helpful, but you should not do them if they increase your pain. If you have a specific back problem such as a prolapsed disk or sciatica, check with your healthcare provider before doing any back exercises.

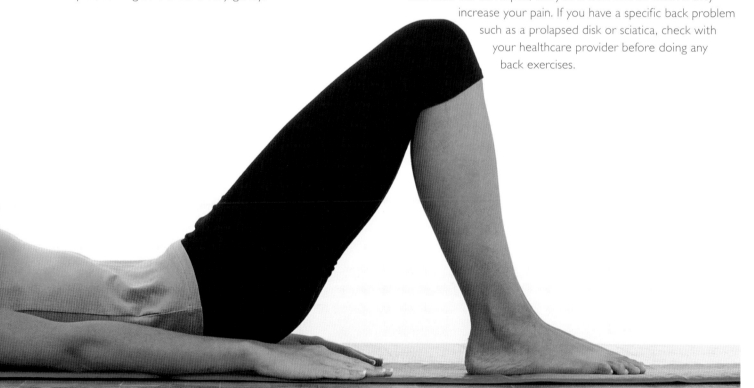

resting an injured back

Your first response to back pain should be to reduce the pressure on the spine and encourage the muscles to relax. Different positions suit different people—experiment to find the one that is most comfortable for you.

position 1

BELOW Lie flat on your back with your knees bent and supported by a pile of cushions so that your hips and knees are roughly at right angles. Alternatively, lie on your back on the floor, but rest your feet on a chair. Support your head and neck if you find it uncomfortable to lie flat.

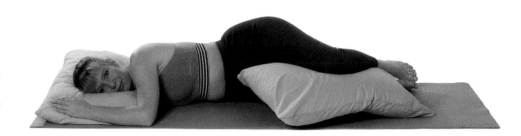

position 2

Lie on your front with a cushion under your abdomen. Rest your head on your hands.

position 3

ABOVE Some people find it more comfortable to lie on their side. Lie with your legs bent and a pillow between your knees to help reduce any strain on the spine. Put another pillow under your head.

tip...

Try to breathe calmly and deeply as you lie down. This will help you to relax.

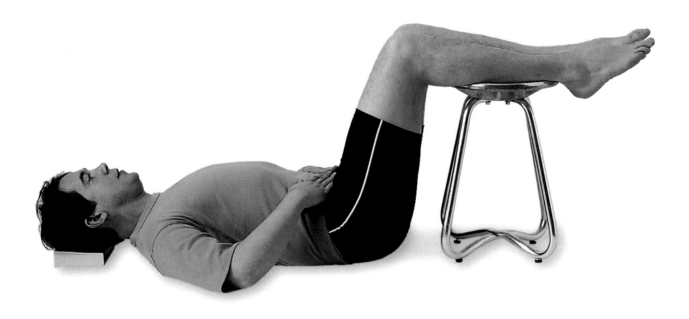

rehabilitation exercises

The following exercises are usually helpful for general lower-back pain.
You can do the lying-down exercises in bed.

first exercises

The following exercises are gentle ones to start with. You should try them only once the pain has subsided enough to let you move about—usually after a day or so. Don't try to warm up first.

as mobility improves

After a couple of days, you can add the following to your routine provided that your mobility is improving. Start by doing only three repetitions at first and gradually build up to ten as you regain your mobility.

Do the exercises three times a day until mobility returns.

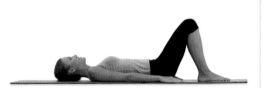

Pelvic tilt
(see page 45)

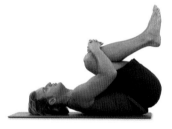

Knee hugs
(see page 46)

Supine twist
(see page 47)

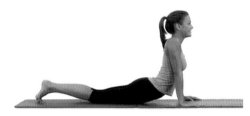

Back arch
(see page 51)

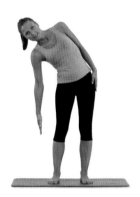

Side bends
(see page 38)

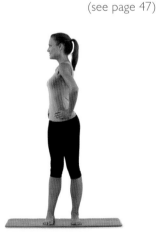

Back twists
(see page 37)

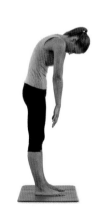

Bending the back
(see page 39)

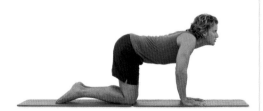

Cat pose
(see page 48)

caution...

These are general exercises. Seek advice from your physician before trying them if you are not sure whether they are suitable for you. Work very gently and stop if you are in pain.

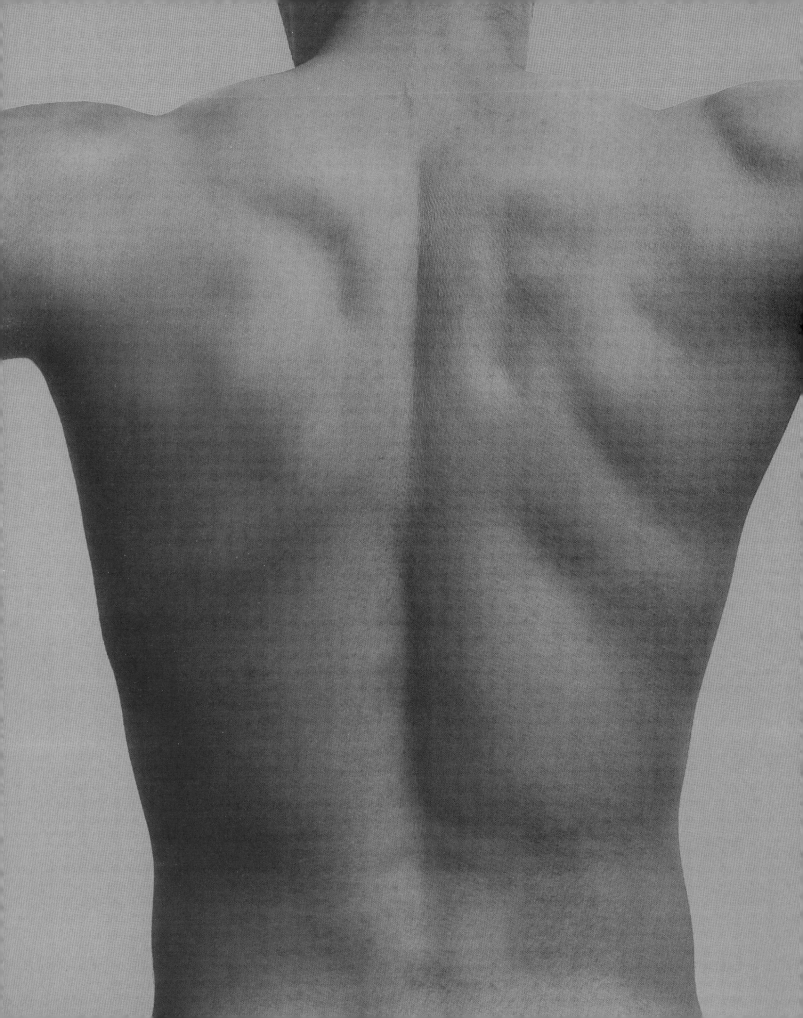

7. helpful therapies

There are many complementary therapies that can help with posture and back problems. Some, such as yoga and the Alexander technique, focus mainly on prevention. Other therapies, including osteopathy, physiotherapy, and acupuncture, can offer a drug-free solution to back pain. Always seek advice from a qualified and registered practitioner, and mention any health issues or treatment you are having. You should also let your physician know about any therapies that you intend trying.

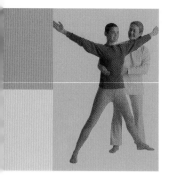

alexander technique

The Alexander technique seeks to re-educate people on how to use their bodies in everyday life. It works on posture, balance, coordination, and breathing, and is completely safe for people of all ages.

If you watch children, you will notice that they naturally hold their heads erect and that they move freely. Most adults, on the other hand, hold themselves in awkward ways, slouching, tensing the shoulders, or thrusting the chin forward. Over time, poor posture becomes a habit: most people are so used to sitting or standing badly that they do not recognize that they are doing it. But these "patterns of misuse" distort the natural alignment of the body, impeding the way that the muscles and joints work as well as the breathing and digestion.

developing awareness

An Alexander technique practitioner works to help you develop greater awareness of the way that you hold yourself and move, so that you can unlearn poor postural habits. Sessions usually take

place on a one-to-one basis. The teacher will observe the way you lie, sit, and stand, and make small adjustments to show you how to improve your posture. You will also practice everyday movements such as answering the phone and ironing, and learn how to perform them without creating tension in the body.

Most people need a course of 20–30 lessons, with regular follow-ups, and it is essential to practice the technique between classes.

who benefits...

Almost anyone can benefit from the Alexander technique, and it is an excellent therapy for improving posture and preventing back problems. It can help to alleviate back pain that is connected to poor posture, and also helps with breathing and stress.

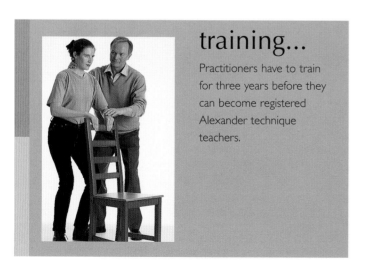

training...

Practitioners have to train for three years before they can become registered Alexander technique teachers.

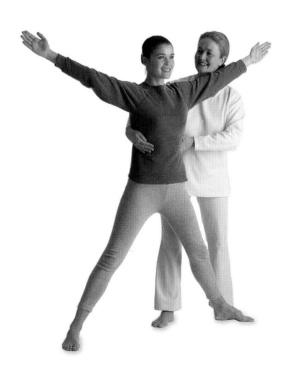

yoga

Yoga is often recommended by doctors as a relaxation therapy, and it can be excellent for improving posture and preventing back problems. It works on the whole body, promoting the mobility of the joints and toning the muscles.

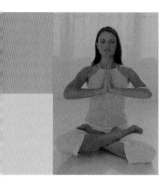

Some exercises can exacerbate an existing back problem or even cause one if done incorrectly. For this reason, it is essential that you find a qualified and experienced yoga teacher and discuss your medical history with him or her. If you have a chronic back problem, seek out a teacher of yoga therapy.

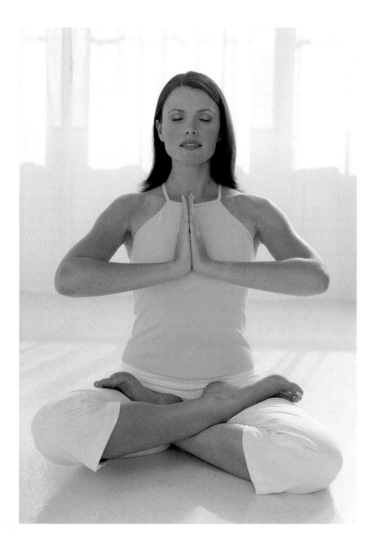

which yoga?

There are many styles of yoga, including:

astanga vinyasa

A vigorous form of yoga that involves doing a set series of postures in a flowing sequence. It is most suitable for people who are young and fit.

iyengar yoga

This yoga focuses on correct alignment and uses props—such as belts and blocks—to help you achieve it. It can be practiced by almost anyone, including those recovering from injury.

viniyoga

Also suitable for people recovering from injury, this is a nondemanding form of yoga that is often taught on a one-to-one basis.

scaravelli

This yoga focuses on working with the natural movement of the spine and body in relation to gravity.

hatha yoga

All the above are forms of hatha (physical) yoga. Classes advertised simply as hatha yoga vary in style but are usually gentle.

caution...

Don't try to push your neck too far when doing yoga stretches. See your healthcare provider for advice before doing yoga exercises if you have a specific neck problem.

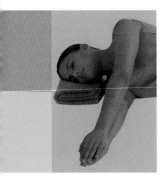

pilates

This is a system of exercise that was developed as a rehabilitation therapy. It is very safe and is suitable for people at all stages of fitness, including those recovering from injuries.

Pilates exercises are done slowly, gracefully, and with control. There is no holding of positions; instead one movement flows smoothly into the next. Central to Pilates is the concept of core strength —strengthening the muscles of the abdomen and back that support your trunk. Teachers stress the importance of pulling in the abdominal muscles and ensuring that the pelvis is in a neutral position before you start to move. Deep, rhythmic breathing and mental focus are also important elements of the practice, which promotes relaxation and concentration as well as physical well-being.

simple but effective

Although the exercises seem very simple, when done correctly they are highly effective in building muscle endurance, strength, and general flexibility. All the muscle groups are worked systematically. Exercises are done on a mat on the floor or on a variety of specialist equipment. Pilates is very good for improving posture. And because it encourages you to develop awareness of the body, you should find over time that you start to move more gracefully in everyday life as well as during the exercises. Pilates is often taught in groups, but one-to-one tuition is usually recommended for people with bad backs or other injuries.

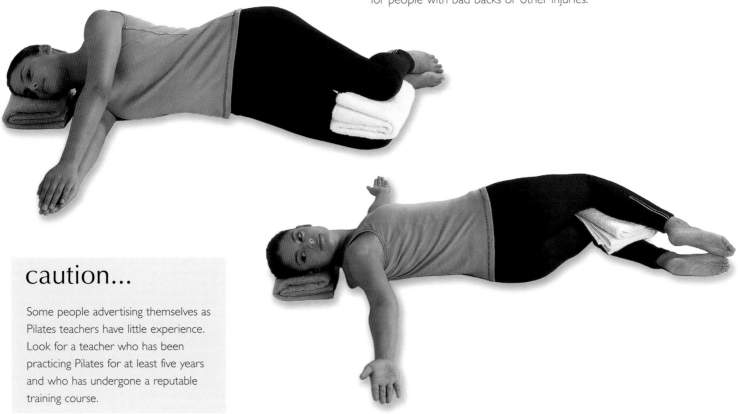

caution...

Some people advertising themselves as Pilates teachers have little experience. Look for a teacher who has been practicing Pilates for at least five years and who has undergone a reputable training course.

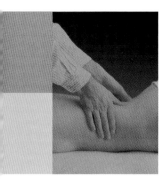

massage

This is an effective way to relax tense muscles. It improves the circulation and helps to flush toxins from the joints and muscles.

There are many forms of massage. The most popular in the West is Swedish massage, which involves a variety of touch techniques to release tension from the muscles and improve the overall functioning of the body. For a full massage, the patient undresses and lies on a special table; oil or talcum powder is usually used to prevent the skin from dragging during the massage. Most therapists can also offer a head, neck, and shoulder massage, which can be given when you are dressed. Some companies enable massage therapists to operate on-site, and this type of massage can be done at a workstation.

The degree of pressure used in massage varies widely. Some therapists use deep pressure, which can be painful, but they should ease off if you find it too much to bear. One particularly intense treatment is Rolfing, a specific therapy that uses firm kneading to release tension from the muscles.

eastern massage

In Eastern forms of massage, such as shiatsu and Thai massage, you remain fully clothed and lie on a mat on the floor. The therapist then moves your body into a variety of yoga-like stretches and uses different parts of his or her body to apply pressure to the soft tissues—for example, the elbows, feet, thumbs, and fingers.

caution...

Training varies widely, so always check that your massage therapist is qualified. Massage may not be suitable for people with certain conditions, such as cancer or osteoporosis—so check with your doctor first.

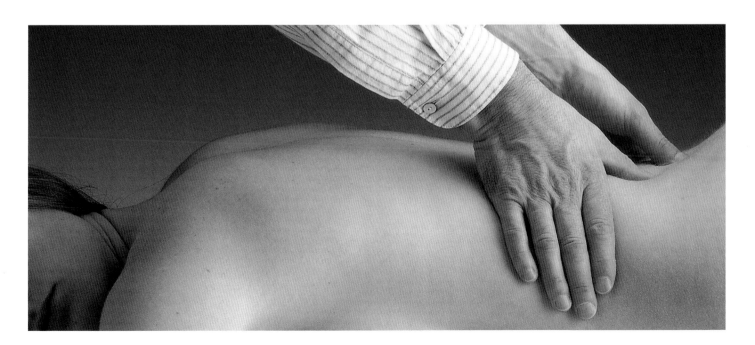

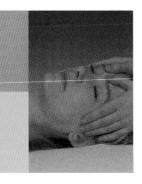

osteopathy

This treatment focuses on the joints and muscles. It is one of the most-used complementary therapies and is highly regarded by many physicians.

Osteopaths believe that the correct alignment of the musculoskeletal system is essential for good health. They use various techniques to improve the alignment and mobility of the joints and soft tissues. These include limb stretches, massage, and vigorous thrusts.

When you visit an osteopath, you will first be asked to stand, sit, and perform a few simple movements. Often you will be asked to undress to your underwear and wear a gown so that the practitioner can see the body's framework more clearly. He or she will also use gentle touch (palpation) to detect points of weakness.

You lie or sit on a special couch for treatment. The techniques should not cause you any pain, but you may hear a popping sound as a joint clicks back into place. Often several treatments are necessary, and you also might be advised to have occasional follow-up sessions. An osteopath might recommend exercises for you to do at home.

cranial osteopathy

Some osteopaths offer cranial osteopathy, which involves making tiny adjustments to the bones of the skull, or cranial-sacral therapy, which focuses on the head and base of the spine. These therapies are very gentle—the adjustments can barely be felt—but are said to affect the flow of cerebrospinal fluid, which bathes the spinal cord and brain.

caution...

Osteopathy might not be suitable if you have a badly prolapsed disk, or a condition such as bone cancer or osteoporosis. Check with your physician whether treatment is suitable for you.

training...

Osteopaths need to complete a four- or five-year training course in order to be allowed to practice.

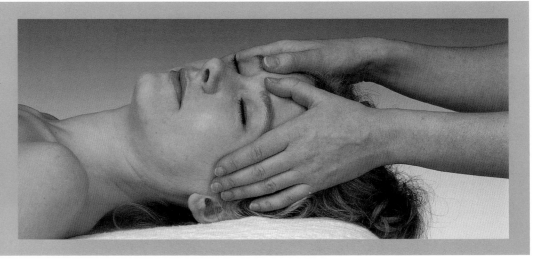

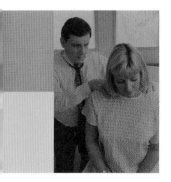

chiropractic

This, like osteopathy, is a manipulative therapy, and the two disciplines share some similar techniques. But while osteopaths focus on improving the mobility of the joints, chiropractics concentrate on the spine.

Chiropractors believe that the spine is crucial to the body's well-being because it houses the central nervous system, which carries messages between the brain and the rest of the body. Since the vertebrae can move, tiny misalignments—called subluxations—can occur. These can interfere with the proper functioning of the nervous system, causing problems elsewhere in the body.

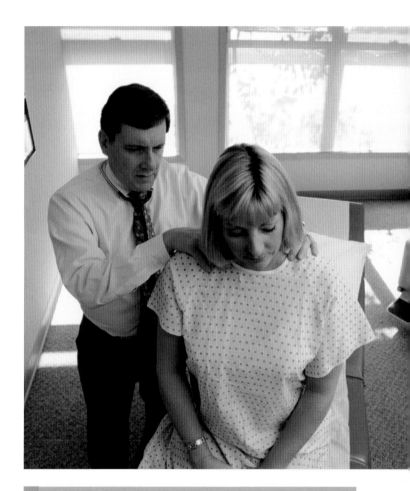

diagnostic technique

A chiropractor will observe you closely at the start of a session and will also use touch to feel for any misalignments in the spine. He or she will gently maneuver your limbs into various positions to check the flexibility of your spine and joints. X-rays are often used to help with diagnosis.

The practitioner will then use various techniques to bring the vertebrae back to the correct alignment: thrusts, massage, stretches, and gentle pressure may be used. Other treatments may also be offered, including hot and cold treatments, ultrasound, and diet and lifestyle advice.

Several sessions are usually necessary. Once the initial problem has been resolved, occasional maintenance treatments might be recommended. After a treatment, you might feel tired, stiff, and achy, so it is important to rest.

caution...

Chiropractic might not be suitable if you have a condition such as bone cancer or osteoporosis, or if you have a badly prolapsed disk. Discuss its suitability for you with your physician.

training...

Chiropractors need to do a three- or four-year course in order to practice.

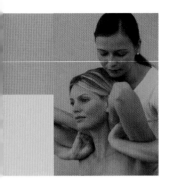

physiotherapy

Physiotherapists usually work with people who have pain and stiffness that has continued for several weeks, and on those with chronic or acute injuries. They use a variety of techniques to improve mobility and reduce pain.

Your physician should be able to refer you to a physiotherapist, or you can find one who works privately. On a first visit, the physiotherapist will observe the way you stand, sit, and walk, and will ask you to carry out a set of simple movements. He or she will also use his hands to feel your back muscles and spine.

Treatment is tailored to the individual. It may include one or more of the following:

● Exercise. The physiotherapist will provide appropriate stretching and strengthening exercises to suit your personal needs.

● Education. The physiotherapist will provide advice on obtaining and maintaining good posture to strengthen and support the spine during activities in the work place, the home, or playing sport.

● Joint mobilization. A technique designed to loosen joints, mobilization involves the slow and deliberate movement of joints through their natural arc of rotation.

● Manipulation. This is a range of techniques used by trained physiotherapists to work on taut muscles and to loosen painful or stiff joints.

training...

Physiotherapists are healthcare professionals who train for three years.

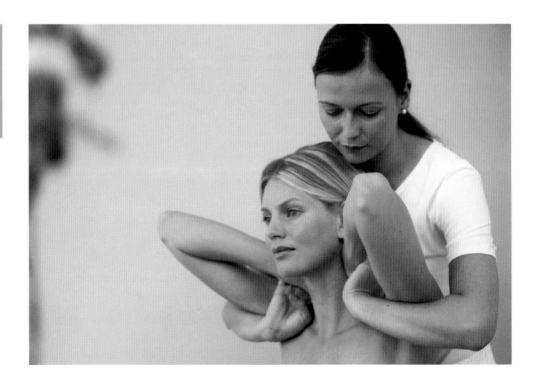

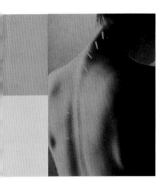

acupuncture

This works on very different principles to Western medicine. However, many physicians now recommend it for pain relief and other problems.

Acupuncture is based on the idea that good health depends on the free flow of energy—called chi—around the body. Fine needles are inserted into specific points on energy pathways (meridians) to release blocked energy and restore a healthy flow of chi.

Numerous research studies have shown acupuncture to be an effective therapy for managing pain and improving general health problems. Western scientists believe that acupuncture works by stimulating the nervous system and blocking the body's pain receptors (so that the brain no longer recognizes the pain is there). As a result, it can be helpful for back problems such as sciatica, wryneck, or muscle tension.

first visit

On a first visit to an acupuncturist, a full medical and lifestyle history will be taken before treatment begins. You lie or sit on a couch for treatment. Several sterile needles may be inserted during a session, and some may be left in place for up to a half-hour. Needling is usually painless, but some points may be particularly tender and so you might experience short-lived discomfort. An acupuncturist might also stimulate points by using finger pressure (acupressure) or heat.

training...

Some doctors offer acupuncture, but may have trained only for a few days. Qualified nonmedical acupuncturists have usually trained for several years.

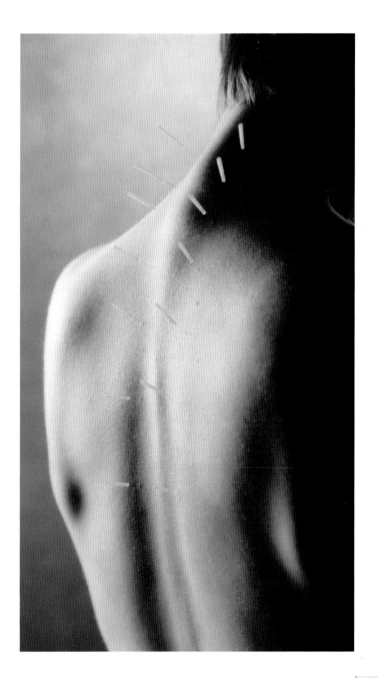

index